The Essential Guide to Avoiding Dementia

understanding the risks

The Essential Guide to Avoiding Dementia

understanding the risks

Mary Jordan

Foreword by Professor Graham Stokes

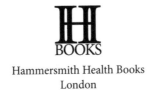

Hammersmith Health Books
London

First published in 2013 by Hammersmith Health Books – an imprint of
Hammersmith Books Limited
14 Greville Street, London EC1N 8SB, UK
www.hammersmithbooks.co.uk

British Library Cataloguing in Publication Data: A CIP record of this
book is available from the British Library.

ISBN (Print): 978-1-78161-016-9
ISBN (Ebook): 978-1-78161-017-6

Commissioning editor: Georgina Bentliff
Designed and typeset by: Julie Bennett
Index: Dr Laurence Errington
Production: Helen Whitehorn, Path Projects Ltd.
Printed and bound by TJ International Limited, UK
Cover image: © Ian Lishman/Juice Images/Corbis

Contents

Acknowledgements

No book is written without help and support from others. *Essential Guide to Avoiding Dementia* is no exception to that rule. I would particularly like to thank Dr Harry Boothby, MA, MB Bch, MRCPsych, who read, corrected and commented upon chapter 2, 'About dementia'; Dr Noel Collins, MB BS (Hons), MRCPsych, who gave me encouragement and answered all my questions patiently; and Dr Gillian Nienaber, BA (Hons), BSc (Hons), CinPsychD, who gave me considerable help with the research into chapter 8, 'Physical and mental illness'.

Thanks are due to Janet Baylis and Andrew Holland, at the Alzheimer's Society's Dementia Knowledge Centre, who gave me an enormous amount of help to find various research papers, on occasion tracking down pieces of research with the minimum of information from me. The Dementia Knowledge Centre is open to anyone via the Alzheimer's Society website and is a great resource for anyone interested in dementia research: www.alzheimers.org.uk/dementiacatalogue.

My friends and family have been very helpful in supplying and giving me permission to use the case history examples and I certainly could not have completed the book without their encouragement, the support of my two sons, Tristram and Rauf, and the many practical suggestions of my daughter-in-law, Erica Arnold.

I would also like to give special thanks to my editor, Georgina Bentliff, who has been a source of great technical support and endless patience.

Preface

What can we do to avoid getting dementia? Whenever I give a lecture or presentation on this disease, this is the question I am most often asked. Any doctor will tell you that to avoid getting a disease it is necessary to know the cause, but at the time of writing we do not know of a specific cause for dementia. Increasingly it is believed that, rather than there being a single cause, it is most likely that there are a number of factors which may predispose us to developing dementia. These are the 'risk factors'; some of these we can modify and some we can take steps to avoid, if we know what they are.

Every day the media runs stories about 'a cure for Alzheimer's disease', but on closer inspection most of these are revealed to be just stories – perhaps with a tiny nugget of information about a new line of research. As I spend my days supporting those with dementia and their carers, it is this research that is of interest to me.

In addition, people like myself who work in the field of dementia-support are able to spend time, so often not available to other health professionals, on in-depth conversation with those whose lives have been affected. We find factors that come up again and again – physical and mental trauma, illness, stress, nutritional habits and lifestyle options.

As I have studied the research and put together information about risk factors, I have begun to notice a number of what I call 'connections'. Many others are interested in these connections too, and in the theories and viewpoints about some of the treatments which have empirical evidence behind them, as well as the hard evidence that comes from medical trials. I have written this book for those people and for anyone who is worried about the possibility of developing dementia.

This book is a review of some of the many areas of research into the risk factors. I discuss some of the conclusions of that research and also look at more tenuous connections which may nevertheless be of interest. I have included case histories where these illustrate important points in the book (these have come from family and friends who have kindly agreed to their inclusion) and I have added a glossary to explain some of the less familiar terms that recur in the book. (You will find these are in bold in the text.) I very much hope the book will stimulate debate and inspire readers to take a look at the original research to which I refer. Most of all, I hope the book will help and encourage anyone concerned with 'dodging the D word'.

Foreword

Mary Jordan writes that dementia is the diagnosis that everyone dreads and recent survey data support this view, that people in middle age and older worry about dementia more than any other condition, including cancer. And this fear coincides with, and is probably influenced by, an anticipated steep trajectory in the number of people living with dementia in the years to come. The outcome will be a doubling of the number in the United Kingdom by 2051, while globally the number will more than treble.

And what causes such extreme worry is that this degenerative and incurable 'politically correct' disease cuts a swathe across society, never respecting power or privilege. Consequently, it is accompanied by a sense, if not a conviction, that nothing can be done to either prevent or reduce the risk of succumbing to a condition that not only results in profound intellectual disability but eventually in the loss of self and of awareness, which can mean that even if your world is supportive, safe and comforting it may be experienced as mysterious, threatening and a source of intolerable insecurity.

In the absence of any realistic hope of a cure, hundreds of thousands of baby-boomers are facing the spectre of advanced dementia. As a result Mary Jordan's book is a timely 'must read'. Embracing dementia awareness, health promotion and risk reduction, this thoughtful and well-written book may just help some avoid the devastating diagnosis of dementia.

Through chapters that are comprehensive, grounded in evidence but accessible to the interested, as well as specialists and practitioners in dementia care, the author explores the myriad of opinions, theories and viewpoints concerning the risks and causes of dementia, some of which surface in the media as sensational claims with only the smallest grain of truth behind them. But then the question is not so much why the media engage in such inaccurate sensationalism as why is it thought that people will be interested in such stories; it is because the fear of dementia is becoming ingrained in the psyche of people in high-income countries across the world.

Surveying the landscape to seek out vulnerability and the possibility of risk-reduction, Mary Jordan considers the potential contribution of physical and mental health, lifestyle, trauma, personality and nutrition, as well as the role of genetics. Her explanations are brought to life by brief case vignettes, while key learning points at the end of each chapter make clear the evidence and arguments.

Throughout, Mary Jordan's message is that we must look at the research: because we do not yet know what triggers the cellular diseases that account for most dementias and so cannot truthfully be sure how to avoid developing, for example, Alzheimer's disease, this book is an honest account of how we can 'lower the odds' in the light of current medical knowledge and experience.

Having considered factors that may make a significant difference to the risk of developing dementia in later life, the book concludes with helpful advice as to what to do if dementia is suspected and how the life of a person living with dementia can be improved through sensible actions and lifestyle changes.

When faced with the mysterious and shocking, people want and deserve knowledge. Without knowledge, fear, insecurity and myth abound. With knowledge comes the prospect of control, appropriate action and the potential for solution. I am in no doubt this book has the potential to change how countless numbers of people might otherwise have ended their lives.

Professor Graham Stokes
Director of Dementia Care, Bupa
Visiting Professor in Person-Centred Dementia Care,
University of Bradford

Chapter 1

Introduction

'Dementia' – it is the diagnosis that everyone dreads. The 'D' word is now more scary than the 'C' word.

You hear things like this said so often:

'As long as I don't go "gaga" I can put up with anything.'

'My Mum was dreadfully ill at the end – but she had all her marbles.'

'Poor dear – he's lost it, you know?'

'She's senile – poor thing.'

Dementia refers to a group of related symptoms that is associated with an ongoing decline in many aspects of the brain and its abilities. The symptoms include problems with short-term memory, mental agility, speech and comprehension. People with dementia may become apathetic; they may lose empathy with others; and sometimes they may have problems with movement and eyesight and experience hallucinations. They may find it difficult to plan things, and to carry out the activities of everyday living.

Dementia is a progressive illness which leads to death. It is not a normal part of aging and only a proportion of people who are old will develop dementia.

The most frightening thing about dementia is that we don't seem to know how to avoid it. You can do your best to avoid a heart attack by exercising and not abusing your body. You can avoid smoking and other carcinogens and hope never to get cancer. You can have your blood pressure tested and take medication to attempt to avoid a stroke. You can keep away from sickness, wash cuts and grazes, and generally avoid infection. You can have a jab against flu and against a myriad of other things which might strike you down and even kill you. But how do you prevent dementia?

Dementia is the ultimate 'politically correct' disease. It can strike whether you are rich or poor, dark or fair, religious or atheist, a nuclear scientist or a road sweeper, a man or a woman, obese or underweight. Current research indicates that age is the biggest risk factor for dementia – and mostly we have to grow old.

The fundamental problem is that we don't yet know what causes dementia – not definitively. Indeed, research seems to indicate that, as with many diseases, there is no one single cause. If you don't know the cause, you can't find the cure, as the saying goes. But is that true?

While we do not know a definitive cause, except in the case of a few relatively rare types of dementia, we do know that there are a number of 'risk factors' which may increase the risk of dementia developing in any one person. It is these, and the large amount of research into causes and risks, that I review through the course of this book.

It is believed that the risk of developing dementia is affected by a combination of genetic and environmental factors. Everyone is at risk, but some of us more so than others. Because a specific cause is not known, it is also true to say that we do not know what factors *do not* cause dementia. However, research indicates that it is not contagious – that is, you cannot 'catch' dementia from being with someone who has the disease.

In this book you will find I sometimes talk about 'dementia' and sometimes about 'Alzheimer's disease'. The two terms are not actually inter-changeable. Alzheimer's disease is just one form of dementia, although it is considered to be the most common. There are probably more than 60 different kinds of dementia. Some of the different types are described in chapter 2, 'About dementia', but some of the research quoted in this book specifically refers only to Alzheimer's disease. To make it clearer, it is possible to have dementia and not to have Alzheimer's disease, but if you have Alzheimer's disease, you definitely have a form of dementia. I have not excluded research which only refers to Alzheimer's disease, because it is likely to have relevance to many forms of dementia.

I have also quoted research originating from many countries. Not everyone uses the same words to describe the same problem. American research, in particular, tends to refer to Alzheimer's disease in a generic way, whereas in Europe the term 'dementia' is used as a global term and Alzheimer's disease is used only for one specific form of dementia. Most of the information we have and most of the research, is concerned with dementia in all its forms.

Not all of the research is conclusive. The medical fraternity holds firmly to the view that nothing is proven unless it has been through the **double-blind trials** (see Glossary) which govern the release of new drugs. As with any disease where the cause and cure are unknown, there are many opinions, theories and viewpoints which would not be considered to be robust evidence because they have not been trialled in this way. I have taken the view that readers of this book may nevertheless be interested in some of these opinions, theories and viewpoints, and in some of the treatments which have empirical evidence behind them. These ideas and viewpoints are not 'evidence based', but people who support those with dementia and their carers come across many 'connections' and cannot help finding them of interest.

The genetic risk

We know that there is sometimes a genetic connection. Dementia, or a pre-disposition to dementia, can run in families, especially something known as 'early-onset dementia'. The three genes that have a major effect on risk of early-onset (that is, younger than 65 years old) Alzheimer's disease are called the 'amyloid precursor protein (APP) gene' and the 'presenilin genes', of which there are two (PSEN-1 and PSEN-2). People with any of these genes tend to develop the disease in their 30s or 40s, and come from families in which several other members also have early-onset Alzheimer's disease. On average, half of the children of a person with one of these rare genetic defects will inherit the disease. It is believed that all those who inherit the genetic defect develop Alzheimer's disease at a comparatively early age. People who do not inherit the disease cannot pass it on. If you have this dementia risk, it is very likely that you are already aware of it as you will have relatives who have developed the condition. This is a rare form of dementia.

It is much more common for people to develop dementia later in life. We all have two copies of another gene – the 'apolipoprotein E (ApoE) gene' – which is implicated in the development of dementia in later life. The two copies may be the same as each other or different, and the variations in combination affect the risk of developing dementia. This is described in more detail in chapter 2. As I explain there, the effect of the ApoE genes seems to be more subtle than the genes affecting early-onset Alzheimer's disease, and even individuals with two copies of the risky form of the gene are not certain to develop Alzheimer's disease. It follows that these genes and their combinations in each individual are not the complete story. As further research takes place more genes are being linked to the risk of developing dementia.

Quite separately, people with intellectual or learning difficulties are more likely to develop dementia than others. In particular, people with Down's syndrome are very likely to develop dementia in mid-life. This has been known only for a relatively short time as it is only recently that people with Down's syndrome have lived beyond mid-life as a general rule. The higher risk of Alzheimer's disease in people with Down's syndrome may be related to the genetic (or rather 'chromosomal') factor behind the syndrome – **chromosome 21**. A protein called 'amyloid beta', which is implicated in Alzheimer's disease (see chapter 2, page 19) is produced from a gene on chromosome 21, and people with Down's syndrome have an extra copy of this chromosome.

Physical and mental disease

We know a lot about 'connections'. There are connections between physical disease and dementia. Some quite rare physical diseases may lead to dementia as a complication of the disease, or sometimes as a progression of the disease. This connection is only briefly covered in this book because the dementia develops as a result of the primary illness and is not a separate disease. However, although there is no absolute proof, there are research papers which seem to indicate connections between a number of physical diseases and the later development of dementia. Of these diseases, the most prominent in the researched evidence is diabetes. Indeed, the evidence of a connection between diabetes and dementia is so well documented and accepted that some scientists even consider Alzheimer's disease to be a third form of diabetes. This is explored in chapter 8.

Other physical diseases are sometimes implicated in the development of dementia in particular cases. The evidence is not always clear enough to indicate that physical disease is the certain cause, but relatives and carers often pinpoint an illness as the beginning of cognitive difficulties, and unofficially many doctors would agree with them.

There are some well-researched connections between some types of mental illness and dementia, and there are some more tenuous connections. I explore these also in chapter 8. Depression seems to be heavily implicated as a pre-cursor to dementia, but it is not completely clear whether the depression is a cause of the dementia or perhaps a result of it. There is a quite a large body of research in this field and it appears that those who have suffered from depressive illness in their past (especially if the depression was difficult to resolve) have a higher than average chance of later developing dementia. Research into connections with other mental illnesses is referred to in this book, but there is much less evidence to support a connection.

Trauma

Many relatives of people with dementia mention that the first intimation that something was awry occurred after a trauma, or injury, physical or psychological. In the case of physical trauma, this can include undergoing surgery. I explore the connection with trauma in chapter 7.

It is known that physical trauma to the head can sometimes lead to dementia. As well as the commonly known **Dementia pugilistica** which results from frequent blows to the head and which can be experienced by boxers and some other athletes, a single head injury may result in dementia, either as an immediate consequence of the injury, or at a later date, although this is certainly not inevitable.

A series of strokes can lead to dementia, and these strokes may not necessarily be major events. A number of small **transient ischaemic attacks** (TIAs) or 'mini-strokes' may lead to what is known as **vascular dementia**. Some doctors think that a vascular 'event' is also what triggers the beginning of Alzheimer's disease.

The effect of psychological stress is more difficult to determine, but there is some research evidence to suggest that psychological stress experienced in childhood may increase the dementia risk in later life. Work-related stress in mid-life has also been implicated as a dementia risk. Post-traumatic stress disorder has been heavily researched, particularly amongst service veterans in the

USA, and the evidence suggests an increase in the risk of developing dementia in those who have experienced significant stress. There is some doubt amongst scientists as to whether stress is a dementia risk (possible cause) in itself or whether the type of person who suffers stress is actually more likely to develop dementia later on. There is a subtle difference.

We do know that stress has a bad impact on anyone who has already been diagnosed with dementia. Such an individual will already be experiencing stress in simply trying to carry out the activities of everyday living. Additional stress in the form of pressure from carers, unexpected events, or the inevitable minor traumas of life, can all seem to make any dementia appear worse. There is also the problem that, as memories are lost and people with dementia start to 'live in the past', stress suffered earlier will resurface and give additional cause for concern.

Lifestyle

Some lifestyle factors are known to increase the possibility of developing dementia in later life. There is some evidence that smoking is a specific risk factor, and the known risks of smoking as a cause of other diseases (some of which are risk factors for dementia themselves) are sufficient to suggest that this is a habit best avoided. The evidence against alcohol is more equivocal and there seem to be definite risk factor differences between light/moderate and heavy alcohol consumption. Other 'recreational' drugs are likely to lead to health problems before dementia may develop.

Nutrition

A great deal of research has been done into whether differing diets make people more likely to develop dementia. Chapter 6, on nutrition, examines this research and you might find some of the actual evidence in this field quite surprising in view of the widely disseminated and commonly believed suggestions that fat is bad for us, that a certain cholesterol level is 'normal', and that our diet should be heavily starch-based. There has also been some significant research into the use of certain food supplements to stave off or to treat dementia. Unfortunately, many initially exciting lines of research, which are often heavily publicised in the national press, have been later found not to bear out their initial promise. Some vitamin supplements may be worth trying, however, as there is some, though limited, evidence to show they are efficacious.

People who have been diagnosed with dementia often suffer from changes in appetite and weight loss. Chapter 6 also suggests how to help these individuals, and how to ensure that they have optimum nutrition despite a possibly varying appetite.

Personality

Many doctors think that dementia tends to develop more frequently in people who have a particular kind of personality and some interesting research has been done in this field. Relatives of those with dementia speak often of a 'personality change', but generally doctors disagree with this idea and suggest rather that dementia emphasises personality traits which are already present and which may have been suppressed or kept to socially acceptable levels in the past. A solitary lifestyle, avoidance of society and an introverted personality type have been implicated in some research, which I discuss in chapter 3.

There are some interesting pieces of research which sometimes seem to contradict each other. For example, having a spouse is said to mitigate against developing dementia, but the spouses of those who have dementia have an increased risk of developing dementia themselves. Contradictions like these are common in research and I endeavour to make some sense of them where possible.

Chapter 1

Positive steps

Chapters 3 to 8 are devoted to risk factors. You may be wondering if there are *any* positive things you can do to prevent or reduce the possibility of developing dementia. The evidence seems to suggest that there *are* lifestyle changes (as mentioned above) and positive actions that you can take. I include these in each chapter and also pull together all the interlinking findings in the final chapter, 'If you are worried you are developing dementia'.

Being flexible

A body of research indicates that, up to a point, level of education makes a difference to the dementia risk. However, all the indications are that the improvement to risk relates to a minimum level of education; the evidence does not suggest that a higher than average education necessarily reduces risk further. There is some empirical and researched evidence, though, that those who have a brain with more 'plasticity' may not manifest the outward signs of dementia even though they have the physical signs in the brain. Plasticity in this respect does not refer to a general idea of high intelligence or education, but to the ability to utilise different areas of the brain, and the willingness to learn new things and accept new experiences. Scientists now believe that some older adults are adept at recruiting additional cognitive resources and that this reflects a compensatory strategy. In the presence of the age-related deficits and decreased 'synaptic plasticity' (see Appendix I, 'The brain – a simple description as it relates to dementia') which accompany aging, the brain manifests plasticity by reorganising its neurocognitive networks. Studies show that the brain reaches this functional solution through the activation of alternative neural pathways, which most often activate regions in both hemispheres (when only one is activated in younger adults). I discuss this research in chapter 4.

We can all make an effort to extend our experiences and knowledge and to do things which are thought to increase the brain's plasticity. The same research into the value of education also frequently covers the effects of social intercourse, experience of life and varied interests and suggests that these factors play an important part in decreasing the dementia risk. At any stage in life we can broaden our horizons, try to extend our social network and take an interest in things around us. Complex things, such as learning a new language, beginning to play a musical instrument or taking up a card game such as Bridge, will all exercise the brain and extend the neural pathways. Even simple activities, such as visiting new places, having interesting conversations or choosing to read a different genre from normal, are thought to be beneficial. Older people often avoid learning or doing new things because it is simply easier to follow old habits. We frequently talk of people being 'stuck in their ways'. If you seriously wish to try actively to avoid dementia you should do your best *not* to be one of those people.

Exercise

As well as exercising our minds, the most positive thing that can be done is to exercise our bodies. Research seems to indicate that physical exercise may even be *more* beneficial than so-called brain exercise in reducing the dementia risk. A number of studies have even suggested that carrying out physical exercise has an effect on brain plasticity. It seems possible that exercise acts directly on the molecular structure of the brain itself and that the beneficial effects are not simply connected with a general benefit to overall health. Some research has indicated that exercise actually strengthens the neural structure, helping the neurons to make connections with each other and thus increasing brain plasticity. It even seems from this research that the number of different *types* of exercise performed is inversely associated with the onset of cognitive impairment. It may be that whilst exercise of any kind is beneficial, the number of different types makes even more difference. It is, of course, possible that taking part in a greater variety of exercise means that people get more social and cognitive stimulation in addition to the beneficial effect of exercise upon the brain – in effect, killing two birds with one stone.

In summary

You may be reading this book because you fear you are in danger of developing dementia; or you may be worried that someone you know and care for is having memory problems and that dementia may be the cause. There is a recognised condition known as **mild cognitive impairment** (MCI) which is now being increasingly mentioned by the medical profession. This is not dementia, but is a condition where some of the features of dementia (mainly memory problems) manifest themselves. It is thought that people with MCI have a higher risk of developing dementia later on. Perhaps you or someone you care for has been diagnosed with this MCI and you are wondering if anything can be done? Generally, if you have this diagnosis, your doctor will not consider it necessary to review your condition at regular intervals and will simply advise you to come back for further tests if your symptoms get worse. There are, however, actions you can take in the meantime that have been shown to be protective. In addition, most of the actions which are thought to reduce the risk of developing dementia are also potentially efficacious in slowing the progress of the disease.

Because we do not yet know the cause of dementia, we cannot truthfully be sure how to avoid developing it. What this book does is explain what the risk factors are thought to be and point to research which suggests how we can 'lower the odds', in the light of current medical knowledge and experience. Each chapter explains how you can modify the individual 'risk factors'. Put simply, if you are worried that you are at risk of dementia, this book explains how you can help yourself. If you are caring for someone with a confirmed diagnosis, then each chapter explains how you can use the knowledge that we do have about dementia to look after this person and improve his/her quality of life.

I hope you find this book useful and pertinent, and I wish you the best of luck.

Chapter 2

About dementia

The word dementia is an umbrella term that is often confused with the more specific 'Alzheimer's disease'. People will say things like: 'My mum had dementia but she didn't have Alzheimer's disease'. This may be perfectly true as there are a number of conditions that may underlie dementia. On the other hand people will say: 'My auntie has Alzheimer's disease, not dementia'. This cannot be a true statement.

There is only a vague perception of what the difference in the meaning of the two terms might be. If you ask any member of the public, you will get replies such as:

'People with Alzheimer's disease become violent.'

'Everyone gets senile dementia as they get older – it's part of the aging process.'

'Dementia is a milder form of Alzheimer's disease.'

'My dad had Alzheimer's disease, but he never developed dementia.'

In fact dementia is a word which describes the symptoms that develop in a number of different diseases. There are more than 60 different kinds of dementia and Alzheimer's disease is only one of them, although it is thought to be the most common, affecting rather more than half of those with symptoms of dementia. The next most common form of dementia is believed to be **vascular dementia**. **Dementia with Lewy bodies** (or 'Lewy body dementia') and **fronto-temporal dementia** are two other types. The term 'fronto-temporal dementia' is used for a range of conditions, including Pick's disease, frontal lobe degeneration and the dementia associated with motor neurone disease. Damage occurs in the frontal or temporal lobe areas of the brain, or both.

Many types of dementia are quite rare. Alternatively, dementia may arise as a result of other diseases (for example, in Huntington's disease).

A condition known as **mild cognitive impairment** (MCI) is now recognised by the medical profession. This is not dementia but is a condition where some of the features of dementia (mainly memory problems) manifest themselves. It is thought that people with MCI have a higher risk of developing dementia later on.

Dementia then, can be described as a collection of symptoms, including memory loss, perceived personality change, and impaired intellectual functions, resulting from disease or trauma to the brain. These changes are not part of normal aging and are severe enough to impact daily living, independence, and relationships.

With dementia, there will likely be a noticeable decline in communication, learning, remembering and problem solving. These changes may occur quickly, or very slowly, over time. If you think someone may have dementia you may have noticed some or all of the following:

- Short-term memory loss
- Impaired judgement
- Difficulties with abstract thinking
- Faulty reasoning
- Inappropriate behaviour
- Loss of communication skills
- Disorientation as to time and place
- Gait, motor and balance problems
- Neglect of personal care and safety
- Hallucinations, abnormal beliefs, anxiety and agitation.

Chapter 2

****

My mother-in-law suddenly became very frightened of being alone in the house. She double-locked all the doors, which at first we thought a sensible precaution. But later we found she had put chairs under the door handles as well to prevent them being opened and she started getting very worried when we left the house and ringing us up at all hours to check where we were.

****

The fact is that many people, as they grow older, experience some of the above symptoms. It is very difficult for someone without medical knowledge to know whether they are a sign of 'normal' aging or evidence of developing dementia. It can be very frightening to forget one's telephone number or some recent event and then to worry that one is developing dementia.

****

Looking back I remember when our first grandchild was born. It was a boy. We were both delighted but for some reason my husband kept referring to the baby as 'she' even though he was called Michael. I dismissed it as a slip of the tongue at the time although he kept on doing it. Now I wonder if that was the first 'sign'.

****

It is possible to compare some of the symptoms and to see how these differ in normal aging and in dementia. For example, any elderly (or not so elderly) person may complain about memory loss but, on questioning, they would be able to provide examples of this, such as: 'I completely forgot where I had put my keys yesterday'. Someone with dementia may not even realise that they have memory problems, may indeed vigorously deny this and may accuse others of making things up when those others give examples of how they have forgotten something.

Most people have occasions when they have to search for a word or substitute a word temporarily. Someone with dementia has frequently to pause to find the right word and may often lose their way in a sentence, perhaps trailing off or diverting to some other subject or drifting into irrelevance.

****

I noticed my sister would lose track of herself in the middle of a sentence. We had always had very lively discussions about many subjects, but she started losing the thread of an argument. If I prompted her she would make an excuse and say I was distracting her or that she couldn't be bothered to talk because she was tired.

****

As we get older some of us may find we have to pause to recall directions clearly or may have to repeat directions to remember them, but we do not get lost in familiar places or forget the route home from the local shops, for example. People with dementia often do get lost in familiar places. Carers often relate that the first sign they noticed was when the person with dementia forgot a simple route, such as the way back from the toilet on a trip out to a restaurant.

Older people generally can remember recent events, especially major events, but people with dementia may forget what happened yesterday, even if it was something important such as a grandchild's christening. They may, however, easily recall events in the far past with great clarity.

****

My father kept accusing us of neglecting him and not coming to see him. If I pointed out that we had come to visit the day before he would strongly deny this and even get abusive. Sometimes I could convince him by showing something I had brought with me on a previous visit but often he would accuse me of tricking

Chapter 2

him or 'planting the evidence' just to catch him out.

****

Older people generally retain their social skills, and normal routines, such as the sequence of events involved in washing or dressing themselves, even if it takes them longer to carry out these actions than when they were younger. People with dementia can sometimes lose interest in social activities or normal hobbies and pastimes and they may forget to wash or be unable to put on a simple article of clothing.

****

The first thing I recall noticing was that he stopped going fishing. Previously it had been his favourite hobby. He often talked about going but he didn't actually do anything. If I asked him about it he usually had an excuse – he was busy, or something had come up which was more important. It was only much later that I looked back and saw that as the first sign.

****

These signs and symptoms are indicative of dementia, but one has to be wary of making assumptions. For example, some forms of depression cause people to lose interest in their appearance and to cease bothering to wash or change their clothes. There are also a number of conditions which may 'mimic' dementia or cause a temporary dementia-like state. One example of this 'delirium' is a low blood sugar level, which can cause susceptible people to become confused and agitated. A urinary infection can also cause similar symptoms to dementia in older people. These symptoms would normally come on fairly suddenly and there would not be the history of a slow decline that we might expect with developing dementia.

Causes of dementia

We do not know an absolute 'cause of dementia'. Research seems to indicate that, as with many diseases, there is no one cause but there are a number of 'risk factors' – both genetic and environmental – which might increase the likelihood of dementia developing in any one person, and which are the primary subject of this book. Our knowledge of these factors suggests that everyone is at risk, but some more so than others. Because a specific cause is not known, it is also true to say that we do not know what factors *do not* cause dementia. However, research indicates that dementia in itself is not a contagious disease – that is, you cannot 'catch' dementia from being with someone who has developed it.

It is important to remember that dementia is *not* a normal symptom of aging. However, age is the most significant known risk factor. It is possible to develop dementia early in life, but the chances of developing it increase significantly as we get older. One in 50 people between the ages of 65 and 70 has some form of dementia, compared to one in five people over the age of 80.

Other risk factors include uncontrolled or poorly controlled diabetes, past trauma to the head, genetic make-up, and some other specific medical conditions.

Certain genes can affect a person's risk of developing Alzheimer's disease, although our knowledge about this is incomplete. The evidence for a genetic cause is clearer for younger-onset than for late-onset dementia.

The genetics of early-onset Alzheimer's disease

The three genes that are thought to have a major effect on the risk of developing Alzheimers disease are:

- the amyloid precursor protein (APP) gene, and
- two presenilin genes (PSEN-1 and PSEN-2).

People with any of these genes tend to develop the disease in their 30s or 40s, and come from families in which several members also have early-onset Alzheimer's disease. The prevalence of these genes is as follows:

- A small number of families throughout the world have a genetic fault on chromosome 21 in the APP gene, which affects production of the protein amyloid. Amyloid build-up in the brain has been linked to Alzheimer's disease.

- A slightly larger number of families carry a fault on chromosome 14 (PSEN-1) causing early-onset familial Alzheimer's disease.

- A very small group of families (mainly in the United States) have a fault on chromosome 1 (PSEN-2), causing early-onset 'familial' (where several generations are affected) Alzheimer's disease.

These risk genes are very rare in the population. Indeed, they account for less than one in 1000 cases of Alzheimer's disease. On average, half of the children of a person with one of these rare genetic defects will inherit the disease. It is believed that all those who inherit the genetic defect develop Alzheimer's disease at a comparatively early age. Those who who do not inherit the disease cannot pass it on.

If you have two or more close relatives (a close relative is defined as a parent or sibling) who developed Alzheimer's disease before the age of 60, you could ask your doctor to advise you about genetic counselling and testing and refer you to a geneticist, if this is thought appropriate.

The genetics of older-onset Alzheimer's disease and vascular dementia

With older-onset dementia the pattern is not so clear. For

example, a gene called **apolipoprotein E (ApoE)** has been shown to play a part in the development of late-onset Alzheimer's disease and vascular dementia. The effects of various combinations of the ApoE gene seem to be subtle and, although it is not believed that these directly cause Alzheimer's, the variations seem to increase or decrease the risk of developing the disease. This gene comes in three forms. Because we inherit one ApoE gene from our mother and another from our father, we each have two copies and these may be the same as each other or different, meaning that each of us can inherit a number of possible combinations. The names and effects of the three variants are as follows:

- ApoE2 – This form of the gene is mildly protective against the development of Alzheimer's disease. Eleven per cent of the population have one copy of ApoE2 together with a copy of ApoE3, and one in 200 has two copies of ApoE2.

- ApoE3 – About 60 per cent of the population have two copies of the ApoE3 gene and they have an 'average risk', which means about half of this group develops Alzheimer's disease by their late 80s.

- ApoE4 – This form is associated with a higher risk of developing Alzheimer's disease. About a quarter of the population inherits one copy of the ApoE4 gene, which increases their risk by up to four times. Two per cent of the population inherit two of the ApoE4 gene – one from each parent – which means they are at 10 times the risk.

As research on the genetics of Alzheimer's disease progresses, researchers are uncovering links between late-onset Alzheimer's and a number of other genes. Some examples are genes called CLU, PICALM, CR1, BIN1, ABCA7, MS4A, CD33, EPHA1 and CD2AP. These genes have a much smaller effect than ApoE on the risk of developing Alzheimer's disease, but research has shown that they may be significant. Such research is very much ongoing and it is possible that new information about genetic risks may become clear in the near future.

There are many rare forms of dementia and some are associated with specific diseases. Usually the disease in question will be identified before any form of dementia develops so this book will not cover these forms of dementia in any detail.

Mild cognitive impairment (MCI)

Mild cognitive impairment, or MCI, is relatively new in medical terminology. It is a descriptive term rather than a specific medical condition or disease. It describes memory loss which the individual and those around them are aware of. Formal memory tests may show up this memory loss but other features of dementia are absent. People with MCI usually have impaired memory but no impairments in other areas of brain function, such as planning or attention span, and no significant problems in carrying out the functions of everyday living.

It is believed that people who have MCI are at an increased risk of going on to develop Alzheimer's disease or another form of dementia. The Alzheimer's Society states that: 'In studies carried out in memory clinics, 10-15 per cent of people with MCI went on to develop dementia in each year that the research results were followed up. In community studies and clinical trials the rates are about half this level, but still represent a significantly increased level of risk'.[1]

Identifying people who have MCI may help them to benefit from early treatment and interventions if they are likely to develop dementia. However, many people with MCI improve or remain stable, and, therefore, do not develop dementia.

Progress of dementia

The progression and outcome of dementia vary, but are largely determined by the type of dementia and which area of the brain is affected. The popular press usually emphasises the loss of short-term memory but, although this is a classic symptom, it may not be the first sign which arouses anxiety in those developing dementia or those around them; emphasis on this aspect may mean that people do not realise that other signs and symptoms may be more important in terms of indicating cognitive decline.

Some people may lose the ability to speak in coherent sentences early on, and this may be the problem which drives them (or drives relatives on their behalf) to seek diagnosis. Loss of this ability may result in long pauses between words, or it may manifest itself in increasing silences and refusal to engage in normal social conversation. On the other hand, the person with dementia may continue to speak quite fluently for a long time but their utterances become confused and muddled and they may seem incoherent to those trying to talk with them.

Sometimes the ability to write is lost quite early on, although coherent speech is retained. Some people may notice that they are no longer able to sign their name. Interestingly, the ability to read (although not necessarily with comprehension) is often retained for many years after the onset of dementia.

The increasing inability to follow a sequence when performing common activities may be what first attracts attention. The person with dementia may find it difficult to follow the correct order of actions when trying to dress themselves, or to make a cup of tea, or to follow a recipe when cooking. Such actions will have been performed for years almost automatically and so when this ability is lost it generally causes great consternation in relatives and family, and will often cause people to visit their doctor to seek a diagnosis.

****

The first indication that there was anything wrong was when my wife found herself in a muddle when cooking. She had always been a great baker of cakes but suddenly it seemed she couldn't understand the recipe and there were several 'disasters' which ended with her in tears before I persuaded her to see the doctor. To be honest I thought it might be something wrong with her sight so the diagnosis was a bit of a shock.

****

In common with the loss of ability to follow a sequence, the loss of orientation may also cause carers and family to be alerted. Sometimes one of the first manifestations is 'getting lost' in a familiar environment or forgetting a commonly used route, such as the way to the local shops. Sometimes this lack of orientation is one of the biggest problems and the person with developing dementia can still hold conversations, carry out common tasks and continue to read and write, but will have difficulty finding their way about.

****

My wife started accusing me of hitting the ball in the wrong direction when we played a game of golf. I didn't realise what she meant at first but within quite a short time I found no one would play with me because I had no idea which way to face when playing. Not long after that I turned the wrong way when leaving the club one night to walk home and if a friend had not chased after me I would have got hopelessly lost even though I only lived a few hundred yards away.

****

Initially the person with dementia is able to cope with normal activities provided they are not over-stressed. Difficulties may only happen occasionally and may be written off by family and friends as the natural 'slowing down' of increasing age. Lapses of memory may be covered up or go unnoticed; difficulties with following a television programme or the plot of a film passed off as due to tiredness; problems with following a sequence of actions (dressing or following a recipe) overcome by taking more time or by preparation, such as laying clothes out the night before. With help and regular support and care, the person with dementia can have a good quality of life, usually for some years.

The disease will progress over time (usually a few years) and there is no known cure. Medication can sometimes stabilise people for a while but (for reasons which are not completely understood) the medication gradually becomes less effective and people with dementia will find that their capabilities deteriorate and their ability to manage life independently disappears. As a general rule, long-term residential care will be needed eventually.

The physical development of dementia

Although the symptoms manifested by dementia are often similar, the early physical effects of the various dementias on the brain and the body are different. Medical science now knows how the disease manifests in the brain, but there is still a lack of knowledge about cause and effect.

In Alzheimer's disease, the two most common features are **plaques** and **neurofibrillary tangles** in the brain. These were first described by Alois Alzheimer, after whom the disease was named. Plaques are small clumps of a protein known as 'beta-amyloid' which usually exists in the brain in a soluble form but in Alzheimer's disease clumps together into solid deposits. These disrupt the normal workings of the brain. During the course of the disease, tangles, which look like dark shapes, develop within the cells of the brain. They are made up of a protein known as 'tau'. This in a normal brain forms rope-like structures which guide chemical messages and brain nutrients down the **axon** of the nerve cells (**neurons**) to send messages on to other cells. In Alzheimer's disease, an abnormal form of tau accumulates which tangles up the rope-like structures. This causes brain cells to die from lack of nutrients. Patients with Alzheimer's also have a deficiency in the levels of some vital brain chemicals which are involved in the transmission of messages in the brain – **neurotransmitters**. Eventually, the brain begins to atrophy. Alzheimer's disease tends to progress steadily, with a slow decline in abilities.

However, some elderly people have many of these plaques and tangles in their brain but they do not display signs of dementia. It is not therefore the 'whole story'.

Vascular dementia develops where problems with blood circulation result in parts of the brain not receiving enough blood and oxygen. We do know that this can cause small areas of the brain to 'die'. Although the human brain can compensate for this (as evidenced by the number of people who recover function after a stroke), if enough areas are damaged so that they can no longer function, the ability to carry out everyday tasks and to learn anything new will be lost. In vascular dementia, progress of the disease is often 'stepped'. Any new event (such as a tiny stroke) will cause an abrupt decline in abilities followed by a period of stability and then a further abrupt decline with each event.

As at the time of writing, medical opinion is changing. The thinking is that even with the plaques and tangles present in the brain, Alzheimer's disease is unlikely to develop without some precipitating factor – most probably a small stroke. This may be small enough to go unnoticed initially, but the disease progresses. For this reason, many doctors now diagnose 'mixed dementia' rather than specifying 'vascular dementia' or 'Alzheimer's disease'.

In **dementia with Lewy bodies**, abnormal structures, known as Lewy bodies, develop inside the brain. These are tiny, spherical protein deposits found in nerve cells. Their presence disrupts the brain's normal functioning, interrupting the action of important chemical messengers, or neurotransmitters, including acetylcholine and dopamine. Researchers have yet to understand fully why Lewy bodies occur in the brain and how they cause damage. Lewy bodies are also found in the brains of people with Parkinson's disease, a progressive neurological disease that affects movement. People who have dementia with Lewy bodies may experience detailed and convincing visual hallucinations (seeing things that are not there), often of people or animals. They are also inclined to fall asleep very easily by day, and have restless, disturbed nights with confusion, nightmares and hallucinations. They may have stiff movements and tremors, faint or fall over, and their abilities are likely to fluctuate daily or even hourly.

In **fronto-temporal dementia**, the frontal and temporal lobes (two parts of the brain) begin to shrink. Unlike other types of dementia, fronto-temporal dementia usually develops in people who are under 65. It is much rarer than other types of dementia. People with fronto-temporal dementia often find that their memory is not affected so early in the disease as with other forms of dementia. Instead, speech may be affected and the social inhibitions which cause us to behave in a considerate manner to others may be lost.

The different types of dementia may manifest differently at first, but all of them are progressive. At present there is no cure and only limited treatment for some types. All bodily functions rely upon the brain to work, and as the brain becomes less and less able to function, so the person with a dementing illness will become less and less able to carry out the functions of everyday living. Eventually, a person with dementia will become unable to walk, to swallow, even to breathe. In actual fact, most people die of an infection or some other illness before this happens.

Medical treatment of dementia

Treatment (where available) is different for the different types of dementia and this is one reason why early diagnosis is so important. Another reason is that, as with any progressive terminal illness, knowledge of the future does allow someone who has been diagnosed to make his/her own plans and indicate personal wishes whilst he/she is still able to do so.

There are medications that can improve symptoms, or temporarily slow down the progression of the disease in some people. The key ones used in cases of Alzheimer's disease are 'cholinesterase inhibitors' and 'NMDA receptor antagonists', which work in different ways.

- Cholinesterase inhibitors include donepezil hydrochloride (Aricept), rivastigmine (Exelon) and galantamine (Reminyl).
- The NMDA receptor antagonist is memantine (Ebixa).

Cholinesterase inhibitors do not work in every case. Between 40 and 70 per cent of people with Alzheimer's disease benefit from cholinesterase inhibitor treatment, but symptoms may improve only temporarily, between six months and a couple of years in most cases. However, new research has indicated that even people with severe Alzheimer's disease may benefit from these drugs. People using these treatments may experience improvements in motivation, anxiety levels and confidence, as well as increased ability to deal with the tasks of daily living, and improved memory and thinking ability. Some people have claimed that the effect is 'like a miracle'; others notice no benefit.

Memantine is licensed for the treatment of moderate-to-severe Alzheimer's disease. It can temporarily slow down the progression of symptoms, including the deterioration in everyday function, in people in the middle and later stages of the disease. There is evidence that memantine may also help behavioural symptoms, such as aggression and agitation.

Trials examining cholinesterase inhibitors for the treatment of vascular dementia indicate that the benefits for this type of dementia are very modest, except in the individuals with a combination of both Alzheimer's disease and vascular dementia (see above). Treatment for vascular dementia is usually concentrated on preventing further vascular problems and may include medication for stroke, high blood pressure, diabetes and heart problems.

There is some evidence that the medications used for Alzheimer's disease are also effective for those who have dementia with Lewy bodies. People who are experiencing symptoms such as rigidity and stiffness may benefit from anti-Parkinson's disease drugs, although these can make hallucinations and confusion worse. For people with dementia with Lewy bodies, neuroleptics (strong tranquillisers usually given to people with severe mental health problems) may be particularly dangerous.

The drugs used for the treatment of Alzheimer's disease do not work for frontotemporal dementia and, indeed, may make symptoms worse. Treatment here is based around support and therapy (such as speech and language therapy).

Other treatments

Much of the treatment for dementia is centred around support. People with dementia can be supported with strategies to manage their declining abilities and these will be offered by community psychiatric nurses, speech and language therapists, occupational therapists and dementia support workers. Carers can be supported by being taught strategies to manage challenging behaviour in those they care for. People with dementia and those caring for them can be directed to relevant financial help and support, aids and appliances to help with daily living, and to suitable day-care facilities, respite care and long-term residential care as required. There is robust evidence to show that good support can delay the need for long-term residential care. The Alzheimer's Society is an excellent source of help and support, and in many cases community mental health teams work with Alzheimer Society Dementia Support workers and Dementia Advisers to provide ongoing support to those who have been diagnosed with any form of dementia, and to those who care for them.

Key points

- Dementia is an umbrella term for the symptoms arising from a number of different diseases
- Alzheimer's disease is one form of dementia
- The symptoms of dementia are different from 'senior moment' memory lapses
- 'Mild cognitive impairment' is not dementia, but may precede dementia
- Younger-onset dementia has a genetic connection
- Dementia has a physical cause – it is not a mental illness
- Dementia is progressive and carers of those with dementia need support.

Reference

1. Alzheimer's Society. *Factsheet 470: Mild cognitive impairment*. 2012: http://alzheimers.org.uk/site/scripts/documents_info.php?documentID=120

Chapter 3

Personality, social behaviours and lifestyle

This chapter looks at behavioural factors that research indicates may affect the likelihood of developing dementia. While there is little that you can do about some factors – for example, an innate liking for, or dislike of, social activity – there is evidence that indicates that some behaviours, such as being socially active, can be a powerful protective factor. This means that a person should not be defeatist about negative risk factors, but should feel encouraged to take steps to counteract them.

Personality traits and the risk of dementia

When carers are talking about a person with dementia they often say things like:
  "His whole personality has changed," or
  "She seems like a different person."
  When a personal history is taken this 'change in personality' may not be so apparent. Indeed, many doctors think that personality type has a great deal to do with the development of dementia.

As we will see, a varied social life, plenty of different interests and mixing with a variety of people as well as a broad education and experience are considered to be protective factors against developing dementia (see chapter 4), but suppose we 'turn this on its head' and consider instead that a person with an outgoing personality, an enquiring mind and a joyful and positive personality is more likely to avoid dementia, despite other predisposing factors being present, than a person who has solitary habits, an introverted manner and a habit of avoiding social intercourse if possible? The first type of person is more likely to have plenty of friends and other social contacts, to have pursued a broad experience of life and to have plenty of varied interests. The second type of person may be a bit of a social recluse, have followed a career in a narrow and specialised area, avoid new experiences and be quite fixed in attitude.

David Snowdon, a neurologist based in the United States, has studied aging and dementia in a population of 678 nuns. 'The Nun Study', as it is known, is a most useful source for researchers because it is a longitudinal study (that is, a study that involves repeated observations of the same variables over a long period of time) of aging and Alzheimer's disease. It began in 1986 as a pilot study looking at aging and disability using data collected from the older School Sisters of Notre Dame living in Mankato, Minnesota, but later expanded to include older Sisters of Notre Dame living in the midwestern, eastern and southern regions of the United States. Participants in the nun study represent a wide range of function and health. Some Sisters are in their 90s; others may be in their 70s. Some of the nuns are highly functional with full-time jobs; others are severely disabled, unable to communicate, and possibly even bed-bound.

Each of the 678 participants in the nun study agreed to participate in annual assessments of their cognitive and physical function. These included medical examinations, giving blood samples and many of the nuns agreed to donate their brains after death for research. This means that this study represents the largest brain-donor population in the world. In addition, the Sisters have given investigators full access to their convent and medical records.

The study has found that personality traits in early, mid and late life have strong relationships with the risk of Alzheimer's disease, as well as the mental and cognitive disabilities of old age. For example, among the documents reviewed as a part of the study were autobiographical essays that had been written by the nuns upon joining the Sisterhood. It was found that an essay's lack of complexity, vivacity and fluency was a significant predictor of its author's risk of developing Alzheimer's disease in old age. Roughly 80 per cent of the nuns whose writing was measured as lacking in 'linguistic density' went on to develop Alzheimer's disease in old age; meanwhile, of those whose writing was *not* lacking, only 10 per cent later developed the disease.[1]

The suggestion that certain personality 'types' might be more prone to develop dementia has been studied elsewhere. A paper published in 2010 detailed the results of a **case-control study** which set out to examine whether personality traits and social networks were significant to the risk of Alzheimer's disease. This study examined 217 individuals diagnosed with probable late-onset Alzheimer's disease (160 women and 57 men). For the purposes of this study, 'informants' who had lived with or were in regular contact with the people studied (the 'subjects') were asked to provide retrospective information about the personality of cases and controls. The controls were recruited from the same population area and were mostly unaffected siblings of the subjects. The informants were asked to remember the subject they knew as she/he had been in their 40s. The subjects were, at the time of the research, aged between 61 and 98 years. Additional assessments were made about social activity when subjects had been in their 40s, and also the level of physical and mental challenge they would have experienced at that time. Cases and controls were also assessed for major depressive episodes and/or abnormal anxiety prior to the age of 50. The results showed that a selection of abnormal personality traits (see below) were over-represented in those diagnosed with Alzheimer's disease (AD). The AD group had a significantly greater number of personality disorder traits compared with the control group. A high correlation was found particularly with cluster-A personality traits (**'paranoid'**, **'schizoid'** and '**schizotypal**') and a lesser but significant correlation with '**dissocial**', '**borderline histrionic**' and '**narcissistic**' traits. In some cases, the differences were particularly striking between those with AD and the controls (for example, some of those who later developed AD had few close friends, found difficulty in enjoying close friendships, bore more grudges, preferred solitary activity, had difficulty expressing feelings and were easily offended). Those people with Alzheimer's disease also had sparser social networks than did controls.

The researchers accepted that the main limitation of the study was that they employed a retrospective rating of personality and social activity so the findings may have been subject to recall bias. However, they concluded that: 'There is an association between abnormal personality traits and AD. Individuals with AD also appear to have had lower levels of social interactivity.'[2]

It is sometimes difficult to distinguish whether apparent personality traits are part of a long history or whether a solitary lifestyle and unwillingness to embrace new experiences are the result of recent life events. Doctors sometimes use a system of asking those closest to the person with dementia to describe his/her personality 10 years previously in order to assess how his/her personality traits might have changed. Of course this is a very inexact method, relying as it does on memory, which may be tainted by past life events and the particular relationship of the relative with the person being assessed. Several questionnaires have been developed to make this assessment, but even the health professionals using them will admit their weakness and lack of objectivity.

There is evidence that the brain is affected by the clinical beginnings of dementia up to 25 years before dementia manifests itself in an obvious way. The brain appears to have a vast 'spare' capacity and it may be that, as evidence seems to indicate, a higher **neural reserve** delays the onset of clinical signs.[3] (See chapter 4, 'Intelligence, education and "expanding the mind"'). What this might mean is that the changes in attitude, activity and what we call 'personality' may begin many years before overt evidence of dementia so that we are once again brought up against the 'which came first?' question.

The five personality factors

The study of personality has a long history. 'Personologists' make much of the innate organisation of personality and believe that behaviour is consistent over time and in different situations. Others ('situationists' or 'behaviourists') assert that the environment and situation may change how we behave. A third view is that of 'interactionists', who believe that people constantly adjust their behaviour according to situations and the society in which they find themselves. Recently, personality psychologists have come to agree on personality traits known as the five factor model consisting of five major personality factors: neuroticism, extraversion, openness, agreeableness and conscientiousness. This model is now so well accepted that any member of the general public can undertake a 'personality test' via the internet and be given scores for these five traits.

Neuroticism is the tendency to experience unpleasant emotions easily, particularly emotions such as anger, anxiety, embarrassment and guilt. Neuroticism also refers to the degree of emotional stability and control of impulses.

Extraversion refers to outgoingness, sociability and the tendency to seek the company of others.

Openness refers to intellectual curiosity and willingness to seek new experiences, appreciate art, be open to new ideas and enjoy variety. Sometimes this factor is called 'intellect'.

Agreeableness refers to the tendency to be cooperative, trustful and compassionate in contrast to being antagonistic and suspicious of others.

Conscientiousness refers to being orderly, dutiful and self-disciplined.

What most personality studies have demonstrated is that personality does in fact remain stable over time. Some investigations have extended into old age (Macrae and Costa 1987[4]; Field & Millsap 1991[5]) and these studies agree with the stability of personality. Where changes do occur they tend to be in agreeableness, which increases, and in extraversion, which declines. In plain words, this might indicate that elderly people become more tolerant but less inclined to socialise.

Personality in dementia

Ann Kolanowski and Ann Whall examined the notion of personality in dementia in a paper published in the *Journal of Nursing Scholarship*. This paper examined personality traits in individuals who had been diagnosed with dementia. As the authors show, research seems to indicate that certain patterns of aberrant behaviour in people with dementia are common according to their past life experiences and how this affected their behaviour pre-dementia. This paper also suggested that the personalities of people with dementia 'reflect adaptive patterns that have served them in the past'.[6]

Generally, it seems that when someone has dementia his/her baseline personal traits do not change; sufferers' personalities reflect the pattern of their past personalities as regards the five factors. So, someone who was introverted and suspicious of others before they developed dementia is not likely suddenly to become outgoing and friendly as a result of their dementia. They are more likely to become more introverted and more suspicious of others. Someone who was generally friendly and trusting will probably remain friendly and trusting.

What often happens, and what carers and relatives often cite as the first signs they notice of a 'change in personality' is that someone who had a previously absorbing hobby stops taking part in it or attending to this hobby. Alternatively, in a similar vein, someone who frequently attended social events and took a full part in them begins to shun going out, or whilst continuing to attend events, takes a less and less active part. Whilst this may seem to be a change in personality trait, it is actually the result of the deterioration in the brain.

The frontal lobe of the brain contains several parts, which all act together to form the 'executive' or 'management' centre. The executive centre is responsible for planning actions and learning new tasks and for motivation and impetus. When this part of the brain is affected, people can lose their 'get up and go', becoming lethargic and unable to perform even regular activities which gave pleasure and satisfaction in the past. It may also be true that someone who is becoming aware that his/her memory and abilities are failing may try to avoid going into situations where he/she feels under stress through having to remember names and faces, or take part in conversations that he/she may have trouble following.

Social interaction and networking

Research cited above also took account of social activity and social networks. A 1999 paper in the *Annals of Internal Medicine* examined the relationship between social disengagement and the incidence of cognitive decline in elderly people living in the community. Altogether 2812 elderly people aged over 65 were interviewed and followed up over several years. Their level of social interaction was assessed by taking account of such things as having a spouse, monthly visual contact with three or more relatives or friends, yearly non-visual contact with 10 or more relatives or friends, attendance at religious services, group membership, and regular social activities. Compared with people who had five or six social ties, those who had no social ties were at increased risk for cognitive decline. The researchers concluded that lack of a good social network is a risk factor for cognitive impairment among elderly people.[7] These conclusions are similar to those drawn by the researchers in the study by Nicholas and colleagues.

One study published in the *Journal of Holistic Nursing* has taken this further and defined 'the six dimensions of wellness' which protect cognition in adults. These six dimensions are defined as follows:

- **occupational**, meaning the ability to contribute to personally meaningful work in a paid or unpaid capacity;
- **social**, meaning the ability to form and maintain positive personal and community relationships;
- **intellectual**, meaning commitment to lifelong learning through continuous acquisition of skills and knowledge;
- **physical**, meaning commitment to self-care through regular participation in physical activity, healthy eating, and appropriate use of health care;
- **emotional**, meaning the ability to acknowledge personal responsibility for life decisions and their outcomes with emotional stability and positivity;
- **spiritual**, meaning having a purpose in life and a value system.

This research looked at such things as the complexity of midlife occupation, marriage, social networks, formal education, intellectual activities, physical activity, healthy nutrition, motivational ability, purpose in life, and spirituality.

The conclusions drawn were that wellness in one or more dimension protected cognition. Cognitive benefits increased if wellness was experienced in more than one dimension. If there was a lack in any one dimension it could be compensated by a higher degree of wellness in another dimension. For example, wide social networks could compensate for unhappiness in one's occupation.[8]

This concept of different dimensions of wellness might suggest why someone with a very fulfilling occupation might find that this 'compensates' for a lack of complex social networks and activities. Sometimes, family members notice dementia symptoms soon after someone has retired, and this theory might suggest a reason, although it would be difficult to prove.

Lifestyle choices and risk of dementia

There are a number of lifestyle choices which are thought to have a bearing on the risk of developing dementia in later life. Some, such as taking exercise and enjoying a varied social life, have been discussed in earlier chapters.

Smoking

Smoking has long been considered to have a detrimental effect on health and some of the research around the effect of a regular smoking habit on cancer and heart disease is now considered to be irrefutable. The evidence for an effect of smoking on the chance of developing dementia has been more debatable. Early research seemed to indicate that smoking actually had a protective effect. This caused some concern in the medical world since at the time of this early research the indications that smoking had a detrimental effect upon other aspects of health were gathering momentum.

Later research, some of which is quoted below, is considered to be more rigorous and have more validity.

In research published in the *Lancet* in 1998, A. Ott and seven colleagues conducted a population-based follow-up study of 'elderly people' who were initially free of dementia. In this investigation, 6870 people aged 55 years and older were classified as 'never smokers' (people who had never smoked), 'former smokers' and 'current smokers'. During follow-up, all cases of dementia were recorded. The study also examined modification of risk by age, sex, and something called the '**apolipoprotein E (ApoE) genotype**' (see chapter 2). Compared with people who had never smoked, this study found that smokers all had an increased risk of developing dementia, including Alzheimer's disease. Smoking was a strong risk factor for Alzheimer's disease in individuals without the 'ApoE 4 allele' (see chapter 2, page 20), but had no effect in participants with this allele. The researchers stated that smoking was associated with a doubling of the risk of dementia and Alzheimer's disease.[9]

Another piece of research, which analysed prospective data from 21,123 people who participated in a survey between 1978 and 1985, looked at the association between mid-life smoking and risk of dementia (Alzheimer's disease and vascular dementia). This study showed that, compared with non-smokers, those smoking more than two packs a day had a much higher risk of dementia – indeed, a greater than 100 per cent increase in risk. However, for those who had given up smoking and for those smoking less than half a pack a day, no increased risk was noted. Significantly, this study particularly concentrated on smoking in mid-life leading to dementia later in life.[10]

It is interesting to contrast the above two papers with a study published in 2000 of 34,439 male British doctors who had been followed up since 1951. This study compared those who had continued to smoke with those who had either never smoked or counted themselves as ex-smokers. (Large numbers of doctors gave up smoking when the evidence that smoking was a major cause of premature death became clear.) Most of the ex-smokers had given up smoking a long time (up to more than 30 years) before this study and so they were considered together with those who had never smoked. Interestingly, this study concluded: 'Contrary to previous suggestions, persistent smoking does not substantially reduce the age specific onset rate of Alzheimer's disease or of dementia in general. If anything, it might increase rather than decrease the rate, but any net effect on severe dementia cannot be large in either direction.' In other words, smoking did not appear to make the onset of dementia arrive earlier as far as this research showed. Indeed, the writers of this paper felt that any effect of smoking on the risk of dementia was negligible.[11]

The research specific to dementia then, is not necessarily conclusive. However, as has been pointed out in previous chapters, there are other physical diseases and events that may well pre-dispose towards dementia. Smoking is known to increase the possibility of being affected by a stroke or developing other vascular disease, both of which are risk factors for dementia. A paper published in 2005 looked at the aggregate risk of various factors in connection with dementia. In this piece of research, 1138 people without dementia were followed up for 5.5 years and the researchers found that four risk factors – diabetes, hypertension, heart disease, and current smoking – were associated with a higher risk of Alzheimer's disease. The risk of Alzheimer's disease increased with the number of risk factors. Diabetes and current smoking were the strongest risk factors in isolation or in clusters, but hypertension and heart disease were also related to a higher risk of Alzheimer's disease when clustered with diabetes, smoking, or each other.[12] If you are keen to avoid the possibility of developing dementia it seems clear that avoiding or giving up a smoking habit is a wise move.

This brings us to another lifestyle habit which is constantly in the health news with often conflicting research results – drinking alcohol.

Alcohol

Before considering research into alcohol intake and dementia it is necessary to refer to one brain disorder which is usually (but not always) associated with heavy drinking and which is sometimes referred to – not totally correctly – as a form of dementia:

'Wernicke-Korsakoff syndrome'. Wernicke's encephalopathy usually develops suddenly. It is due to a lack of thiamine (also known as vitamin B1). People who drink excessive amounts of alcohol are often thiamine deficient because of poor eating habits and because alcohol can interfere with the body's ability to convert thiamine into the active form of the vitamin. There are three main symptoms: involuntary, jerky eye movements or paralysis of muscles moving the eyes; poor balance, staggering gait or inability to walk; and drowsiness and confusion. If treated in time, by injections of thiamine, the symptoms are usually reversed in a few hours. However, if Wernicke's is left untreated, or is not treated in time, brain damage may result and Korsakoff's syndrome may develop. This results in short-term memory loss, changes in personality and attempts by the sufferer to make things up to fill the inevitable memory gaps. Treatment for Korsakoff's syndrome consists of complete abstention from alcohol and injections of thiamine. Generally, someone who has developed Korsakoff's syndrome does not make a complete recovery but this treatment will prevent a deterioration of the condition. Sometimes this condition can result from poor nutrition without alcohol intake, but this is rare in the western world.

The evidence for alcohol intake as a risk factor for the development of dementia is, if anything, even more confusing than that concerning a smoking habit.

Research conducted as part of what is known as the 'Rotterdam study', published in the *Lancet* in 2002, looked at the drinking habits of 7983 people aged 55 years and older. This study concluded that compared to complete abstinence, light to moderate alcohol consumption was associated with a reduced risk of dementia in older adults. No variation in the protective value of any particular type of drink was noted.[13] 'Light to moderate' drinking was defined as one to three drinks per day.

One noted limitation of this study is the fact that levels of alcohol consumption were self-reported. There is a general belief within the medical profession that people under-report both the amount they smoke and the amount they drink.

The researchers in this study suggested that the beneficial effects of low to moderate alcohol consumption might have been because of a reduction in cardiovascular risk factors. Alternatively, they might have resulted from a direct effect on cognition by the neurotransmitter acetylcholine being released in the part of the brain called the **hippocampus** (see page 163). Acetylcholine is known to facilitate learning and memory. It is thought that a low concentration of alcohol stimulates the release of acetycholine whereas higher concentrations inhibit this. Such an effect would suggest that heavy drinking increases the risk of dementia.

A review of research into connections between alcohol intake and dementia by Luc Letenneur of the Université Victor Segalen in Bordeaux, published in 2004, [14] included reference to the above study and also to a well-known study conducted in France by researchers (including the author of this review) which specifi- cally looked at wine consumption and risk of dementia. Subjects were visited at home by a psychologist and several characteris- tics were recorded, including wine consumption. In this study moderate drinking was defined as three to four glasses of wine per day. A first analysis showed that moderate wine consump- tion was associated with a lower risk of 'incident dementia' three years after the initial visit. When considering Alzheimer's disease, mild drinkers and moderate drinkers had a significant decrease in risk. Another analysis confirmed these results after adjustment for many other potential confounding factors. This French study concluded that moderate drinking of alcohol was associated with a reduced risk of dementia. [15]

Letenneur's review also considered several similar studies conducted in other parts of Europe and pointed out that the benefits of moderate alcohol intake seemed to be confined to men over the age of 40 and women over the age of 50. In younger people, the consequences of alcohol consumption are more negative due to accidents and diseases directly linked to alcohol. This review suggested that the elderly should not be discouraged from drinking alcohol but concluded that it would be premature 'to advise people who did not drink to start drinking' in order to avoid developing dementia.[14]

More recently, two studies were presented at the Alzheimer's Association International Conference in Vancouver. These found that moderate alcohol consumption later in life, heavier alcohol consumption earlier in life, and binge drinking later in life increased the risk of declining cognitive performance.

The first study, by Tina Hoang and colleagues of NCIRE/ The Veterans Health Research Institute, San Francisco, and the University of California, San Francisco, was conducted only on women. Being a conference report rather than a journal article, it leaves some questions about methods and analysis unanswered, but the findings are interesting nonetheless. It followed more than 1300 women aged 65 and over for a period of 20 years. The results showed that women who had drunk greater amounts in the past and subsequently reduced their drinking had a 30 per cent increased risk of cognitive performance decline. Participants who drank moderately (defined as 7-14 drinks per week) in the later phases of the study were approximately 60 per cent more likely to develop cognitive impairment and women who changed from being non-drinkers to drinkers over the course of the study increased their risk of developing cognitive impairment by 200 per cent. The researchers concluded that alcohol intake in later life might not be beneficial in women.[16] Compare this with the study above suggesting that moderate alcohol intake seemed to benefit women over the age of 50.

The second study analysed data from 5075 US adults aged 65 and older over eight years. Cognitive function and memory were assessed using telephone interviews, and results showed that those who reported binge drinking (four or more drinks in one sitting) twice a month were more than twice as likely to experience a higher level of cognitive decline.[17] This study, of course, has the same limitations as the Rotterdam study in that the amount of drink consumed and the incidence of binge drinking were self-reported.

Whatever might be concluded from the state of current research into alcohol consumption as a risk factor for developing dementia in later life, we do know that alcohol consumption has a bad effect on anyone who already has dementia. This is obvious really. Even those of us who have no cognitive impairment have more difficulty in solving problems, carrying out complex tasks and driving a vehicle after consuming alcohol. If the brain is already under stress and cognitive performance is impaired, it would hardly seem sensible to administer a substance likely to make things worse! However, it is worth bearing in mind the advice given in chapter 9 on what to do after a diagnosis. In general, people are happier and keep their quality of life longer if they continue to enjoy leisure pursuits which they took part in before the diagnosis. If you or the person you are caring for enjoyed a gin and tonic before dinner or a pint once a week there is probably no harm in continuing this if your doctor agrees. However, bear in mind that memory problems may mean that someone with dementia forgets that they have had a drink so that one drink may become one drink after another without supervision!

Caring for someone with dementia and the risk of developing dementia

This chapter on personality and lifestyle seems an appropriate place to mention an interesting and unusual piece of relevant research. In 2010, Maria Norton and colleagues published a paper in the *Journal of the American Geriatric Society* which investigated whether spouses of people with dementia were at an increased risk of developing dementia themselves. The high level of stress experienced by spouse caregivers is well known and it is equally well known that stress has an effect on cognitive functions. However, rather than looking at stress in general, this research specifically investigated the risk to the spouse caregiver of later developing dementia. The authors found that spouses of those with dementia had a 600 per cent greater risk of dementia than spouses of people without dementia. They reported a 'clear increased risk of incident dementia among older adults whose spouses have dementia'.[18]

This seems like quite a frightening finding and might make some people question the accepted conception that you cannot 'catch' dementia from someone who has it. However, as the authors pointed out, there might be several explanations for the finding of a greater risk in spouses. As far as possible the researchers themselves tried to adjust for socioeconomic status, and for environmental factors, such as a healthy or less healthy lifestyle shared by both spouses. However, it is possible that a shared lifestyle at least partially explains the findings. There are likely to be similarities in terms of diet, exercise pattern and personality type which increase the risk of dementia for both partners. Dementia in one partner leads to social isolation for both and social isolation is a major risk factor, as we have seen. Caregivers are also more likely to be depressed and to have less time to exercise or follow a hobby or interest of their own, and these too are potential risk factors for dementia (see chapter 8 on mental health).

The authors were also careful to make the point that, while the overall risk for dementia among married individuals whose spouse had dementia was high, many spouses were not affected.

Conclusion

Scientific research is divided on the effect of personality traits on the likelihood of dementia development. The evidence concerning other lifestyle choices is also not completely clear-cut.

However, in the interests of reducing risk it would seem wise to avoid smoking (or to give up the habit), to keep to a moderate alcohol intake and increase our social networks, seeing friends, enjoying various activities and taking an interest in life generally.

Key points

- Some research seems to indicate that certain personality types are more at risk of dementia
- Existing personality traits tend to become more pronounced in dementia
- Lifestyle choices such as a smoking habit or heavy drinking of alcohol may increase dementia risk
- A broad social life and good social networks decrease the risk of dementia

References

1. Riley KP, Snowdon DA, Desrosiers MF, Markesbery WR. Early life linguistic ability, late life cognitive function, and neuropathology: Findings from the Nun Study. *Neurobiology of Aging* 2005; 26(3): 341-347.

2. Nicholas H, et al. Are abnormal premorbid personality traits a marker for Alzheimer's disease? A case-control study. *International Journal of Geriatric Psychiatry* 2010;25(4) :345-351.

3. Stern Y. Cognitive reserve and Alzheimer's disease. *Alzheimer Disease and Associated Disorders* 2006; 20(2): 112-117.

4. Macrae RR, Costa PT. Validation of the five-factor model of personality across instruments and observers. *Journal of Personality and Social Psychology* 1987; 52(1): 81-90. DOI: 10.1037/0022-3514.52.1.81

5. Field D, Millsap RE. Personality in advanced old age. *Journal of Gerontology* 1991; 46(6): 299-308.

6. Kolanowski AM, Whall AL. Life-span perspective of personality in dementia. *Journal of Nursing Scholarship* 1996; 28(4): 315-320.

7. Bassuk SS, Glass TA, Berkman LF. Social disengagement and incident cognitive decline in community-dwelling elderly persons. *Annals of Internal Medicine* 1999; 3: 165-173.

8. Strout KA, Howard E. The six dimensions of wellness and cognition in aging adults. *Journal of Holistic Nursing* 2012; 129-136.

9. Ott A, Slooter AJC, Hofman A, Harskamp F van, Witteman JCM, Broeckhoven C van, Duijn CM van, Breteler MMB. Smoking and risk of dementia and Alzheimer's diseases in a population-based cohort study: the Rotterdam study. *Lancet* 1998; 351: 1840–1843.

10. Rusanen M, Kivipelto M, Quesenberry CP, Zhou J, Whitmer RA. Heavy smoking in midlife and long-term risk of Alzheimer disease and vascular dementia. *Archives of Internal Medicine* 2011; 171(4): 333-339. DOI: 10.1001/archinternmed.2010.393

11. Doll R, Peto R, Boreham J, Sutherland I. Smoking and dementia in male British doctors: prospective study. *British Medical Journal* 2000; 320; 1097-1102.

12. Luchsinger J et al. Aggregation of vascular risk factors and risk of incident Alzheimer's disease. *Neurology* 2005; 65(4): 545–551.

13. Ruitenberg A et al. Alcohol consumption and risk of dementia: the Rotterdam study. *Lancet* 2000; 359: 281-286.

14. Letenneur L. Risk of Dementia and Alcohol and Wine Consumption: a review of recent results. *Biological Research* 2004; 37: 189-193.

15. Lemeshow S et al. An illustration of analysis taking into account complex survey considerations: the association between wine consumption and dementia in the Paquid study. *American Journal of Epidemiology* 1998; 148: 298-306.

16. Hoang T et al. 20 year alcohol consumption patterns and cognitive impairment in older women. Presented at Alzheimer's Association International Conference 2012.

17. Laing I et al. Heavy episodic drinking and risk of cognitive decline in older adults. Presented at Alzheimer's Association International Conference 2012.

18. Norton MC et al. Increased risk of dementia when spouse has dementia? The Cache County study. *American Geriatric Society* 2010 ; 58(5): 895–900. DOI: 10.1111/j.1532-5415.2010.02806.x.

Chapter 4

Intelligence, education and 'expanding the mind'

Many people equate lack of intelligence with the development of dementia. However, as we will see, the connections between intellectual level and the risk of development of dementia are complex. Whilst it is known that people with an intellectual disability have a greater risk of developing dementia as they age, above a certain level a person's raw intelligence level doesn't appear to be a significant risk factor. (An IQ of 70 to 75 is regarded as 'borderline intellectual impairment' according to the AAID (see below).) Someone with a 'high IQ' is not necessarily at a lower risk. However, the level of education achieved does seem to make a difference, along with variety in life experiences, the breadth of social experiences and contacts, and the continued pursuit of activities which stimulate and expand the mind.

I will address these more general issues very shortly, but will begin by looking at the more specific subject of intellectual disability, and especially of Down's syndrome where there seems to be an important genetic factor.

Intellectual disability and the risk of dementia

'Intellectual disability' is defined by the American Association on Intellectual and Developmental Disabilities as: 'a disability characterized by significant limitations both in intellectual functioning (reasoning, learning, problem solving) and in adaptive behavior, which covers a range of everyday social and practical skills. This disability originates before the age of 18.'[1] It does appear that people with intellectual disabilities have a greater risk of developing dementia as they age than others. This does not mean that all people with intellectual disabilities will suffer from dementia, but if they do, they generally develop it at a younger age than others.[2] This may not always be recognised because the standard diagnostic tests for dementia are difficult to apply in cases of intellectual disability and the initial symptoms may be different.

Down's syndrome

A higher risk and the possibility of earlier development of dementia is particularly the case for people with Down's syndrome. It is now believed that one in three people with Down's syndrome develops dementia in their 50s, and it is thought that more than half of those with Down's syndrome who live to be 60 or over will develop the condition. The most common form of dementia experienced by people with Down's syndrome is Alzheimer's disease,[3] although some may develop other forms of dementia.

Until recently it was rare for people with Down's syndrome to live beyond middle age and the additional problem of an increased tendency to develop dementia was not understood or recognised. The reason Alzheimer's disease is more common in people with Down's syndrome is still not completely known, but we do know that it is associated with increased production of a protein called **amyloid beta**, which forms hard insoluble plaques in the brain. As amyloid beta accumulates it is thought to cause loss of brain cells (**neurons**), although exactly how neuron loss occurs is also not well understood. The higher risk in people with Down's syndrome may be related to **chromosome 21**, because amyloid beta is produced from a gene on chromosome

21 and people with Down's syndrome have an extra copy of this chromosome.

It may also be that the age when the symptoms of Alzheimer's disease actually develop are related to a person's mental capacity (**'cognitive reserve'**) or some anatomic characteristics of the brain. I discuss more fully below the possibility that people with more brain cells (neurons), and connections between neurons, and more education may not develop symptoms as early as people with less cognitive reserve. People with Down's syndrome may develop symptoms of Alzheimer's disease earlier in life than other people because of both their increased production of amyloid beta *and* their smaller cognitive reserve.

It is known that people with Down's syndrome often show different symptoms from the common ones associated with the early stages of dementia and may experience more rapid progress of the condition. It seems they are in general less likely to receive a correct or early diagnosis. The clinical picture of Alzheimer's disease with Down's syndrome is complex because of the pre-existing cognitive impairment. Someone with Down's syndrome may have relatively unsophisticated social skills and difficulty in communicating with others, and this can mean that they are unable to present their symptoms verbally or at all.

Generally it seems that memory problems are less likely to be the first sign of developing dementia in someone with Down's syndrome. Personality changes, such as a more stubborn attitude or the tendency to become angry or withdrawn, are more likely to be the first signs.[2] If the person with Down's syndrome begins to have epileptic fits *which they were not prone to before*, this is also a specific indication of developing dementia. Carers, particularly carers in an institutional setting, may have difficulty in discerning that symptoms are not typical for someone with Down's syndrome and may attribute behavioural changes to the learning disability and not to developing dementia. (One term for this is 'diagnostic overshadowing').[4]

This may mean that referral for a diagnosis is made later than would normally be the case. Where someone with Down's syndrome is living within his/her own family, relatives may notice unusual symptoms, but even if they draw these to the attention of medical staff, their concerns may be dismissed and alterations in behaviour attributed to the learning difficulty and increasing age.

Even after a diagnosis has been made, there are likely to be further difficulties. Those with Down's syndrome may not be able to understand the diagnosis. However, as I have explained in other chapters, this lack of understanding is true of many people who do not have a learning difficulty at the time of a dementia diagnosis simply because of the nature of the disease (see chapter 2).

It has been reported that Alzheimer's disease in those with Down's syndrome presents with a greater prevalence of low mood, excessive activity and restlessness, disturbed sleep and increased uncooperativeness.[4] One common symptom is to become much more upset by changes to routine than was previously the case. This need for routine and difficulty with changes to timetables is common to nearly all the dementias, but is of course also linked to personality traits (see chapter 3).

Given this pattern, people with Down's syndrome who develop dementia will require very specific support to understand the changes they are experiencing and to access appropriate services after diagnosis, and as dementia progresses. In addition to the difficulties in communication which often manifest with dementia, there may be additional problems because sometimes those with Down's syndrome are already using other forms of (possibly) non-verbal communication due to speech difficulties. Other learning difficulties may make it impossible for information literature to be accessible or for the intervention of clinical staff to be accepted.

On the plus side, people with Down's syndrome may already

be in a supported living environment, where they are given help to allow them to live independently. When the staff in the supported living facility feel able to cope, then, as with any case of dementia, the continued stability and safety of the familiar environment are vitally important for the person with developing dementia. Staying in a familiar environment with familiar carers reduces confusion and fear in the person with Down's/dementia and the value of being able to continue to live in the environment they know until the end of life is huge. In some cases, care staff may not feel that they are trained to cope with the combination of Down's syndrome and dementia. It can be very traumatic for someone to have to move from a familiar environment at a time when he/she is probably feeling less able to cope than usual, more fearful and more confused. It is also difficult to find new residential facilities that can cope with the combination of behavioural symptoms which result from Down's syndrome and dementia together.

Where someone with Down's syndrome is living in the family environment, the family will need extra support and may find it particularly difficult and feel very guilty if (as is likely) a move to a residential care home becomes necessary. Support services specifically catering for people with Down's syndrome and dementia are sparse. Carers and families of someone with Down's syndrome who develops dementia should remember that the Alzheimer's Society will support them in the same way that they support anyone else who has, or is caring for, someone with dementia. Families and carers are also entitled to the same help from NHS and social care agencies as the carer of someone without Down's syndrome who develops dementia.

An interesting piece of research looked at the *mothers* of Down's syndrome children. Those who had given birth to a Down's syndrome child before the age of 35 were found to be at a higher risk of developing Alzheimer's disease than mothers who gave birth to children with other forms of learning disability. To be more precise, mothers who were under 35 years of age when their children with Down's syndrome were born were four to five times more likely to develop Alzheimer's disease than mothers in the control group. For mothers who were over 35 years of age when their children with Down's syndrome were born there was no significant increase in risk. There did not appear to be any increased risk among fathers of Down's syndrome children.[5]

Other intellectual disabilities

Some studies suggest that people with intellectual disabilities other than Down's syndrome are also at a higher risk of developing dementia and that they also may exhibit initially symptoms other than memory impairment.[2] There is still only rather limited research in this area.

Autism/Asperger's syndrome

People who care for someone with dementia often report a lack of empathy as one of the first noticeable symptoms. Carers who have a relative or friend with autism or Asperger's syndrome sometimes note that the lack of empathy and inability to sympathise with, or seem to understand the concerns of, others has similarities with the behaviours of those with autism / Asperger's.

D K Sokol and colleagues, in a research paper on autism, Alzheimer's diseases and fragile-X syndrome, highlight the genes which are implicated in both autism and Alzheimer's disease.[6] However, little more significant research seems to have been done concerning any connection between these two disorders. It should be noted that autism is defined as a disorder of neural development characterised by impaired social interaction and communication, and by restricted and repetitive behaviour. Autism affects information processing in the brain by altering how nerve cells and their synapses connect and organise themselves, but how or why this occurs is not well understood.

There is to date no indication that someone with autism or Asperger's syndrome is at higher risk of developing dementia. It may be, however, that those with autism/Asperger's are less likely to be diagnosed even if they develop dementia because their condition is not easily understood.

Education

As I noted at the start of this chapter, a person's raw intelligence level doesn't appear to be a significant factor in determining the chance of developing dementia. However, the level of education achieved does seem to make a difference to the level of risk, along with variety in life experiences, the breadth of social experiences and contacts, and the continued pursuit of activities which expand the mind.

The exact level of education that makes a difference is not precisely known, but evidence seems to indicate that any protective factor may be due to education creating a higher 'neural reserve', which delays the onset of clinical signs. In other words, education, by developing the brain, gives the brain more capacity for making connections, retrieving memories and using vocabulary. This means that even when some parts of the brain may be degenerating due to some form of dementia, other parts may be called into use to 'get around' the problem.

We know that something like this happens with stroke victims. If someone has suffered a stroke, a part of their brain effectively 'dies' and is no longer of use. However, people who have had a stroke can relearn abilities they have lost. They can recover lost functions through structural changes in the surviving brain cells (or 'neurons'), or by learning new ways to solve old problems. Put simply, people recover lost functions by 'educating' a different part of the brain to form new connections and neural pathways.

It may be that if, in early dementia, a part of the brain fails to function, then a similar process takes place. It seems that someone who has benefited from more than basic education has so developed their brain that it is able to 'get around' the problems of lost connections by changing its pathways, in the same way as a motorist might use a diversion to avoid a road closure.

The conclusions of research into the benefits of education are not always clear. Research results have appeared to show differences depending upon the type of measure of cognitive ability which have been used in the research. Where researchers have used a test called the 'Mini Mental Status Examination' (MMSE), a commonly used test in determining the progress of dementia, then a higher level of education has appeared to show a protective effect. For example, in one research project in the USA, Constantine Lyketsos and colleagues tested a group of 1488 people on three occasions over a period of 11½ years. They observed that more education was associated with less cognitive decline. Having at least eight years' education was associated with the maintenance of cognitive function during aging. However, beyond nine years, education was not associated with a further reduction in cognitive decline.[7]

On the other hand, where researchers have tested individual elements of cognition, results have not always been so clear cut. For example, Christensen and colleagues reported that whilst education affected general mental status and verbal abilities (such as extent of vocabulary), it did not seem to affect speed of processing in a group of older people tested over a 3.6 year period.[8] They suggested that education had a 'compensatory' rather than a protective effect. This might tie in with the theories of brain plasticity and cognitive reserve which we will examine shortly.

An interesting study that was mainly involved in observing the effect of education in early-onset Alzheimer's disease and **fronto-temporal dementia** looked at 44 people with dementia who were under 65 years and used the number of years of formal education as a marker for **cognitive reserve** (see below). The findings of this study suggested that education played a part in upholding 'attentional' capacity. In other words, formal education helped those with dementia to better retain the ability to pay attention. Given that a short attention span is a major problem in early stage dementia, this research is significant.[9]

Scientists and researchers talk about 'cognitive reserve' and 'brain plasticity' and in order to follow how these factors may affect the risk of dementia we need to understand what they are and what we can do to influence them.

We know quite a lot about the development of the brain in infancy. In the early years the brain develops its 'links'. A newborn's brain is only about one-quarter the size of an adult's. It grows to about 80 per cent of adult size by three years of age, and 90 per cent by age five. This growth is largely due to changes in individual neurons (brain cells), which are structured much like trees. Each brain cell begins as a tiny 'sapling' and gradually sprouts hundreds of long, branching **dendrites**. Brain growth is largely due to the growth of these dendrites, which serve as the receiving point for input from other neurons. **Synapses** are the connecting points between what is called the **axon** of one neuron and the dendrite of another. While information travels down the length of a single neuron as an electrical signal, it is transmitted across the synapse through the release of tiny packets of chemicals, or **neurotransmitters**. On the receiving side, special receptors for neurotransmitters change the chemical signal into an electrical signal, repeating the process in this next neuron in the chain. The number of synapses in the cerebral cortex peaks within the first few years of life, and then declines by about one third between early childhood and adolescence.

The initial perception of an experience is generated by a subset of neurons firing together. Because they have fired together once, the neurons involved are more inclined to fire together in the future. This is known as 'potentiation' – recreating the original experience. If the same neurons fire together often, they eventually become permanently sensitised to each other so that if one fires the others do as well.

Thought processes are complex. We may describe an action in a 'straight line' fashion, but in fact each thought process involves many neurons and many synaptic connections. If one connection fails, several others may still function. Take the example of a leaf. It grows on a tree, it is green, it rustles in the wind, it may have a name which reminds us of something else (Ivy and Holly are common girls' names and we also connect them with Christmas), it evokes a season of the year (spring, summer or autumn), it may have a scent and so on. Let us suppose that we pick up a leaf and for the moment we cannot recall what kind of a tree it comes from. It is prickly and reminds us of Christmas and the face of our little niece comes to mind. Of course – it is a holly leaf. The direct 'connection' from seeing the leaf to remembering its name momentarily failed but by using other connections the brain has led us to the name of the leaf. Thought processes are like that.

It is believed that education enables the brain to develop its ability to make these various 'connections'. Take the simple example of the leaf again. If we lived in an oak wood and never left it, if the only trees we ever saw were oak trees and we were brought up in an environment where the only leaves we saw were oak leaves, then the first time we saw a holly leaf we might not recognise it as a leaf. Formal educational experience, and exposure to a variety of other experiences, hobbies, activities and events, develop our ability to extend our brain connections.

Brain reserve

The idea of a 'reserve' in the brain comes from the observation scientists have made from post mortem examinations that some people whose brains showed extensive physical signs of Alzheimer's disease (amyloid plaques, neurofibrillary tangles, etc), in life had no, or very little, manifestation of the disease. Reserve is perceived as having both passive and active components. Passive components are structural, or anatomical, features of the brain. Active reserve is taken to mean the efficiency of the neural networks and the brain's ability to compensate or use alternative networks after an injury, such as, a stroke. Dr Yaakov Stern in his paper 'Cognitive reserve and Alzheimer's disease' suggests similarly that the concept of cognitive reserve may take two forms. In 'neural reserve', the existing brain networks are more efficient or have a greater capacity to resist damage. In 'neural compensation', other brain networks may compensate for the networks that are damaged.[10]

The scientific world is still not certain whether cognitive reserve actually prevents dementia or whether the ability to 'redirect' our brain connections just prevents the manifestation of dementia symptoms. Either way, it does not matter to the average person who is trying to avoid dementia. Since we are normally unaware of attempts by our brain to make use of 're-directions' in neural pathways, the non-appearance of signs of dementia is good enough. As far as your neighbour is concerned, if you don't show signs of dementia, you don't have it.

The brain's ability to change and develop

Neuroplasticity or 'brain plasticity' refers to changes in neural pathways and synapses which are due to changes in behaviour, environment and neural processes, or changes resulting from bodily injury. Education, although considered important, is thought to be just one factor responsible for increased brain plasticity. Exposure to a range of activities and experiences seems to be equally important.[1] As I explain in chapter 3, people who develop dementia often have a long history of avoiding social-ising, having few friends and acquaintances and tending to be introspective 'loners'. Sometimes they have been wrapped up in their career, and their work has seemed to give them all the social contact they wanted. The carer may give a story of a person who, whilst perhaps enjoying family life, chose not to have a large social acquaintance, enjoyed one or two hobbies, most likely of an isolated nature (for example, stamp collecting, fishing), but who has gradually dropped the practice of these hobbies and who now resists going anywhere new or into strange situations. Other dementias develop differently and the same pattern may not be apparent in, say, vascular dementia or fronto-temporal dementia. Often relatives of someone in the early stage of Alzheimer's disease suspect that depression may be to blame for the loss of interest in society and life events, and, as discussed in chapter 8, depression may often be a contributory factor.

As we get older many of us find it more difficult to learn new things. Many elderly people rely on their children to set up a new electrical device, such as a DVD player, after it has been purchased, or they refuse to learn how to use a computer, or retain an old power tool when a newer one would be more efficient because they are 'used to' the old one and know how it works. Sometimes people return again and again to the same holiday destination, use only familiar shops, always fill the car at the same garage, always take the same route when driving to visit others. Research has shown that older people are just as capable of learning new things as younger people, although they may take more time to learn a new skill, so this is not the reason for this unwillingness to try new things. It is thought possible that the learning process may be slower because an older person already has so many 'filed' memories. The brain is getting full of stored information. However, healthy older people can usually learn new things well even if it takes a little longer than when they were young. It is the diseases connected with aging, not the aging process itself, that affect mental agility. If an older person is not depressed and if he/she is interested and assuming there is no disease (like Alzheimer's disease) present, new ideas can be just as appealing and new skills just as well acquired in old age as they are in youth.

So it would seem that older people avoid learning or doing new things because it is simply easier to follow old habits. It is as if our brain automatically routes us towards the methods, the abilities and the directions which we already know and it would take a big effort to change our ways.

It may also appear pointless to make such an effort. If we have found that one way of doing something works best for us, what, we may ask, is the point of trying another? As for setting up the DVD recorder, well our child (or our grandchild) can do it so much more quickly than we can so why not ask them to help? If we have found the perfect holiday destination, why make the effort to go elsewhere? And of course we only use that particular petrol filling station because it is on the way home and so convenient. Yes, the one two streets away is cheaper but not enough to make it worth the effort to change our ways. As for learning another language, or taking up a new hobby – it's too late at my age! You can't 'teach an old dog new tricks'.

Resistance to change

One of the noticeable effects of dementia is how it may seem to change someone from being amenable to being awkward.

****

My cousin's wife has dementia and he says the most difficult thing is the isolation. He says that they receive invitations but at the last minute his wife will refuse to go out. So they are invited to fewer and fewer occasions and go out less and less. He says sometimes he is desperate for company but that even though his wife when asked will agree that it would be nice to see 'so and so' she will always refuse to leave the house at the last minute.

***

My husband used to enjoy eating out. Now, however, he refuses to go out to a restaurant and even demands that we eat the same boring menu at home. He has a range of dishes he will accept and if I serve up anything else he becomes grumpy and sometimes won't eat.

****

Examples like those in the box are more likely to indicate a desire for safety and security on the part of the person with dementia rather than a 'change in personality'. The fact is that when dementia affects the brain it becomes more difficult for someone to do anything new or different. If we consider what is involved we can understand why. To try to learn or to attempt something different involves our brain in following new and different 'pathways'. As we have seen, the well-used pathways in the brain become more entrenched each time we carry out a previously enacted action. The neurons are used to firing together. As we grow older we tend to do the same things in the same way. We do this because it is easier for us. For someone with dementia (in whom some neurons have probably degenerated) it is even more difficult to plan or attempt to carry out any new action. The easiest thing to do in this situation is to refuse to do anything which takes us away from the well-worn path with which our brain can still cope. When asked to do something which might involve a measure of thought or effort, the simplest thing to do is to refuse.

You may think there is a world of difference between being a bit 'stuck in our ways' and someone with dementia refusing to accept any variation in the daily pattern, or becoming upset and confused when challenged by a change in routine. Or you may consider that it is but a short step from one to the other. Either way, it is of immense benefit to the active brain to keep challenging it with attempts to learn new things, to find new ways to carry out familiar tasks, and to avoid normal routines becoming unchangeable habits.

We already know quite a lot about how **cognition** changes as we age: our ability to process information becomes less efficient, including our speed of processing, working memory capacity, inhibitory function and long-term memory. However, our implicit memory, knowledge storage and verbal ability are resistant to aging and are protected from age differences. You may question how we are able to learn new things as we age if the above findings are true. It has been suggested that the aging brain develops a 'compensatory scaffold'.[12] The idea is that the brain recruits extra circuitry that shores up the declining structures whose functioning has become less efficient. To illustrate this idea we might consider the skill acquired when learning to drive a car.

Many of us can remember our driving lessons, which may have begun with the feeling that there were far too many things to remember and coordinate (gear stick manoeuvres, steering, braking, watching the road, anticipating obstacles, etc) and proceeded through a nervous acquisition of skill (learning to reverse around a corner) to confidence when we realised that we were in control of the car. Over a period, the mechanical skills of driving become ingrained in us so that we no longer think of putting our hand on the gear-stick before we engage the clutch. This action seems to happen automatically. If we see an incident or an obstacle ahead, we engage our feet, hands and brain in a coordinated action which enables us (hopefully) to come to a controlled stop or to engage in an evasive manoeuvre. We do not need to think about doing these things; our brain reacts instinctively and engages the body in the correct actions (foot on the brake pedal, hand on the gear lever) without our being conscious of this activity. So we have 'learned' to drive, and driving is no longer an effort.

What we have, in effect, been doing is engaging and developing a set of neural circuits to provide structure for the performance of the new task. After a while the performance of this task (driving) no longer required such an effort. Our circuitry has shifted and we have honed an optimal circuit of neural regions that are interconnected and make for efficient processing and action. However, it is suggested that the structure, or 'scaffold', which we developed whilst learning the new skill of driving does not disappear. It remains available as a secondary 'ready' circuitry which can be called upon when required, for example, if for some reason the skill of driving becomes once more a challenge.

The 'scaffold' theory suggests that as we age and as some brain functions become less efficient we once more invoke the 'scaffolds' which were set up during the learning process, to help us perform familiar tasks and cognitive functions which become more of a challenge due to failing neural circuitry. This means that when we are required to learn new processes in older life, our brains are still capable of making the effort required to do so. However, different areas of the brain, and perhaps different processes, are involved than when undergoing a similar learning process when younger.

A study led by the Rotman Research Institute in Toronto has found that older adults can perform just as well as young adults on visual, short-term memory tests. What the study found, however, was that older adults used different areas of the brain than younger people. Ten young adults (aged 20 to 30) and nine older adults (aged 60 to 79) participated in identical visual, short-term memory tests while their brain activity was measured using an imaging technique called 'positron emission tomography' (PET). PET acts as a marker to show which brain areas are lighting up during a memory performance task. Results showed that young and older participants performed the memory task equally well, but the neural systems or pathways supporting performance differed between young and older individuals. While there was some overlap in the brain regions supporting performance (for example, occipital, temporal and inferior prefrontal cortices (see

Appendix 1 – The brain)), the neural communication between these common regions was much weaker in older individuals. Older individuals compensated for a weakness in neural connections by recruiting unique areas of the brain, including the **hippocampus** and dorsal prefrontal cortices. The hippocampus is generally used for more complicated memory tasks.[13]

Putting theory into practice

The research I have quoted here and in other chapters clearly indicates that learning new things, enjoying a variety of new experiences, and keeping a varied social life and acquaintance, are factors that may make a significant difference to the risk of developing dementia in later life. How do we put this knowledge into action?

Remember that the emphasis should be on variety; on fresh, new and different experience. So doing more of the same crosswords and number puzzles that you already enjoy is not the answer. To a certain extent you should put your brain under stress – a good stress, the kind that is experienced when learning something new. However, we none of us want to make life a chore and there is a pleasant comfort in familiar things. What you should try to do is to make sure that you do not drift into the 'comfortable' kind of life that happens when every day is predictable, every experience a repeat of that which happened yesterday. It is a good thing sometimes to re-examine our routines and to decide which ones serve a purpose and which are just comfortable grooves.

- Why not buy a different newspaper today?
- Why not try shopping in a supermarket you do not usually patronise?
- Why not walk to the shops instead of driving – or drive instead of walking – or maybe catch the bus?
- Why not experiment with a different recipe for lunch?

- Why not experience the taste of a piece of fruit you have never tried?

If you can do these simple things, you can make advances in your behaviour patterns. If you love classical music, try listening to some jazz now and again, or, failing that, to some composers whom you might not normally patronise. If you don't play an instrument you could try to learn to play one. Listening to music and playing music and singing all activate areas of the brain which help us with other functions. So good is singing thought to be as a therapy in dementia that the Alzheimer's Society even has a specific service labelled 'Singing for the brain', though a 'Conchrane Review' of all published research concluded that there is as yet no reliable evidence that music therapy helps with dementia symptoms. Maybe you think you can't sing? The most modern theory is that virtually everyone has 'a voice' and can be trained to produce a melodic sound. There are teachers who specialise in giving individual lessons to people who would like to sing but have never had the courage to try. You don't have to join a choir. Why not take a few lessons? Similarly you don't have to learn to play an instrument to an especially high standard. You could play just for pleasure at home.

Have you ever tried to paint, or are you someone 'without an artistic bone in your body'? You don't have to paint a portrait to have a new experience in the artistic world. You could paint a mural. Or paint on the garden fence if you are afraid to sully the house walls. There is nothing to stop you painting over your mistakes, after all. Maybe you could try wood carving? Or origami? Why not try to throw a pot? If the logistics seem too complicated (potter's wheel, kiln, etc) buy some modelling clay and start with that. I know a keen gardener who modelled individual clay 'caps' for her garden canes, painted and varnished them and discovered in herself a new hobby which later turned into a paying business.

It is never too late to learn a new language. Bilingual people are known to be less likely to get dementia and it is thought that the learning of a second language stimulates an area of the brain which helps to improve mental health. Research by Ellen Bialystok and colleagues, published in 2007, looked at the effect of bilingualism on maintaining cognitive functioning and delaying the onset of symptoms of dementia in old age. On average, those people who were bilingual showed symptoms of dementia four years later than those who spoke only one language. Those who were bilingual and who did develop dementia showed the same rate of decline in **Mini-Mental State Examination** (MMSE) scores over the four years subsequent to the diagnosis, indicating that once diagnosed the bilingual people kept their four-year advantage.[15]

You could also open to yourself a whole new area of pleasure by finding new literature to read in your second language, listening to radio programmes broadcast in your second language, being able to do without sub-titles on films and being able to speak to the locals in their own language when you go abroad on holiday.

You could have some fun by setting a new challenge every day. Try to write out the whole alphabet with your non-dominant hand. Complete a word puzzle which you never usually attempt. Eat porridge for breakfast instead of cold cereal. Get a grandchild to teach you a computer game. Send someone an electronic birthday card. Learn how to use an application on your mobile phone which you never usually bother with. Plan and plant a flowerbed. Learn how to say 'Good morning' to your Chinese neighbour in his own language. Learn a poem. Play a game of chess.

Stimulating the brain in early dementia

If we accept that a certain level of education, a varied social life and new experiences might reduce the risk of dementia, is there any indication that giving cognitive stimulation might help those with **mild cognitive impairment** (MCI) or who are in the early stages of dementia? Most dementia support staff would certainly agree that this is so. Day centres for people with dementia are not there just to give the carer a rest, although this is an important and not under-rated function. Good day centres set out to provide cognitive stimulation in the form of enjoyable activities, discussions and reminiscence, quizzes, crosswords, number puzzles and games. Carers report that the person they care for enjoys the day centre and seems brighter (although possibly tired) after his/her time there.

Research supports the idea that cognitive stimulation helps to retain and even improve cognitive abilities. Glenn E Smith and colleagues published a paper on their research into whether a cognitive training programme based on the principles of brain plasticity made a difference to memory and attention span. The training used a brain-plasticity-based computer training programme and involved people using the programme for one hour per day, five days a week for eight weeks. The experimental programme improved generalised measures of memory and attention more than a computer programme used as an 'active control' that was not designed to stimulate brain plasticity.[16]

However, what may help a healthy individual may be too much for someone with dementia, even in its early stages. It is important not to deluge a person with dementia with 'brain training' tasks or force him/her to feel constantly under pressure to perform. Someone with dementia will have slower thinking processes, but that does not mean to say he/she is stupid. He/she will generally just need more time. You should do your best not to put the person you care for under stress and this means you should not be constantly 'testing' him/her. Nor, contrary to what you might think from what I have written above, should you force him/her into new experiences or confuse him/her with too many new faces or visits to strange places – it is a question of degree, and what the individual is still capable of. As far as possible, you should help the person you care for to continue to enjoy the hobbies and social life he/she has previously known. It is important to allow more time for preparing to go out, and for everyday routines. As far as possible, allow the person you care for to manage tasks for him/herself whilst he/she still can, and as time goes on, with the minimum of help which will allow him/her to still feel a sense of achievement from completing tasks.

It is good to introduce new experiences and people into the life of the person you are caring for provided it is done at a pace he/she can cope with. For example, as time goes on you might need someone to help you, perhaps by assisting the person with dementia with personal care, or by keeping him/her company when you have to be absent. Introduce new ideas and new faces gently, and allow time for acclimatisation, and always ensure that the person with dementia feels secure with the new activity or company.

Cognitive stimulation is a good thing if carried out without adding to the stress which someone with dementia is already experiencing just by living his/her everyday life. If the person you care for is offered any cognitive stimulation programme by local professionals from the Community Mental Health Team, then it is worth taking advantage of this. If day-centre care is suggested, do not dismiss this because of a mistaken idea that it is 'baby minding' or that by accepting it you are failing in your duty. You will be acting in the best interests of the person you care for.

The future

There is still much research to be done in the area of intelligence, education and brain plasticity in connection with the risk of developing dementia. However, the current level of research indicates that a good basic education, a varied social life and a mixture of interests and experiences are all important elements in improving the chance of avoiding dementia in later life.

Key points

- Raw intelligence does not in itself seem to protect against developing dementia
- Level of education does seems to have some bearing on risk
- Intellectual disability, and Down's syndrome in particular, are associated with a much higher relative risk
- Early symptoms of dementia in Down's syndrome are hard to pick up and diagnosis is often delayed
- **Brain plasticity** and **cognitive reserve** may be factors in the risk of developing dementia
- Variety in life, in social contacts and in leisure pursuits all seem to be significant factors
- The brain changes with age but dementia is not a natural result of aging
- People with dementia enjoy brain-stimulating activities in a safe and non-threatening environment

References

1. American Association on Intellectual and Developmental Disability: http://www.aaidd.org/content_104.cfm
2. Strydom A, Livingston G, King M,Hassiotis A. Relevance of dementia in intellectual disability using different diagnostic criteria. *British Journal of Psychiatry* 2007; 191: 150-157 DOI: 10.1192/bjp.bp.106.028845.
3. Fact sheet: Learning disabilities and dementia. Alzheimer's Society website. www.alzheimers.org.uk/site/scripts/documents_info.php?documentID=103
4. Levitan GW, Reiss S. Generality of diagnostic overshadowing across disciplines. *Applied Research in Mental Retardation* 1983; 4(1): 59-64. dx.doi.org/10.1016/S0270-3092(83)80018-6

5. Schupf N, et al. Specificity of the fivefold increase in AD in mothers of adults with Down syndrome. *Neurology* 2000; 57: 983.

6. Sokol DK, et al. Autism, Alzheimer disease, and fragile X: APP, FMRP, and mGluR5 are molecular links. *Neurology* 2011; 76(15): 1344–1352. DOI: 10.1212/WNL.0b013e3182166dc7

7. Lyketsos CG. Cognitive decline in adulthood: an 11.5 year follow up of the Baltimore Epidemeological Cachement area study. *American Journal of Psychiatry* 1999; 156: 58-65.

8. Christensen H, et al. Education and decline in cognitive performance: compensatory but not protective. *International Journal of Geriatric Psychiatry* 1997a; 12: 323-330. DOI: 10.1002/(SICI)1099-1166(199703)12:3<323::AID-GPS492>3.0.CO;2-N

9. Fairjones SE, et al. Exploring the role of cognitive reserve in early onset dementia. *American Journal of Alzheimer's Disease and Other Dementias* 2011; 26(2): 139-144.

10. Stern Y. Cognitive reserve and Alzheimer's disease. *Alzheimer Disease and Associated Disorders* 2006; 20(2): 112-117.

11. Nicholas H, et Al. Are abnormal premorbid personality traits a marker for Alzheimer's disease? A case-control study. *International Journal of Geriatric Psychiatry* 2010; 25(4): 345-351.

12. Park DC, Reuter-Lorenz P. The adaptive brain: aging and neuro-cognitive scaffolding. *Annual Review of Psychology* 2009; 60: 173-196. DOI: 10.1146/annurev.psych.59.103006.09365

13. McIntosh AR, Sekuler AB, Penpeci C, Rajah MN, Grady CL, Sekuler R, Bennett PJ. Recruitment of unique neural systems to support visual memory in normal aging. *Current Biology* 1999; 9(21): 1275-1278.

14. Koger SM, Brotons M. Music therapy for dementia symptoms. *Cochrane Database of Systematic Reviews (Online)* 2000(3):CD001121].

15. Bialystok E, Craik FIM, Freedman M. Bilingualism as a protection against the onset of symptoms of dementia. *Neuropsychologia* 2007; 45: 459–464.

16. Smith GE, et al. A cognitive training programme based on principles of brain plasticity: results from the Improvement in Memory with the Plasticity-based Adaptive Cognitive Training Programme (IMPACT) Study. *Journal of the American Geriatric Society* 2009; 57: 591-603.

Chapter 5

Exercise

There is a large body of evidence which suggests that physical exercise not only prevents the development of dementia but also slows the rate of decline in people who are already diagnosed with the condition. We are all familiar with the constantly re-iterated mantra that 'exercise is good for you', and most of us take this for granted, but perhaps we should examine why this is considered to be so and especially why physical exercise is said to be of such benefit to the brain.

Most advice to exercise more emphasises the benefits to the cardiovascular system. One medical internet site suggests that the health benefits of regular exercise include:

- up to a 35% lower risk of coronary heart disease and stroke
- up to a 50% lower risk of type 2 diabetes
- up to a 50% lower risk of colon cancer
- up to a 20% lower risk of breast cancer
- a 30% lower risk of early death
- up to an 83% lower risk of osteoarthritis
- up to a 68% lower risk of hip fracture
- a 30% lower risk of falls (among older adults)
- up to a 30% lower risk of depression as well as a 30% lower risk of dementia.[1]

Exercise is known to have multiple positive effects in older adults, including those with disabilities. In particular, exercise prevents and reduces the risk of developing secondary conditions that arise from functional decline and lack of physical use. Physical exercise is a considered to be a primary and secondary preventer of cardiovascular illness, particularly that due to ischaemic heart disease. Regular physical exercise is thought to implement its beneficial effects through reducing the incidence and severity of obesity and the consequent risk of type 2 diabetes; improving glucose tolerance; the prevention of the development of blood clots and the lowering of blood pressure. (Glucose tolerance and the part this plays in the risk of dementia related to diabetes is discussed in chapter 8.)

It is thought that low physical activity roughly doubles the risk of coronary artery disease and is a major risk factor for stroke. As well as the direct physical benefits on the body's cardiovascular and metabolic parameters, exercise also provides benefits through reducing the effects of stress, ameliorating and preventing depressive illness and anxiety in those who are at risk of, or suffering from, cardiovascular disease, and through improvements in self-esteem.

The evidence that physical exercise has a beneficial effect on the cardiovascular system is now considered incontrovertible. A healthy cardiovascular system protects against the development of vascular dementia. Vascular dementia, as previously explained, is caused by problems in the supply of blood to the brain. Typically, the symptoms of vascular dementia begin suddenly, sometimes following a stroke. Vascular dementia also tends to follow a 'stepped' progression, with symptoms remaining at a constant level for a time and then suddenly deteriorating. Sometimes no precipitating stroke is recognised but when a history is taken carers can recall a time or an incident from which symptoms seemed to stem. Often the cause is a so-called 'mini-stroke' (a transient ischaemic attack, or 'TIA' for short).

Occasionally carers will not be able to pinpoint a precipitating event and will maintain that the loss of cognition has happened slowly and almost imperceptibly. In such cases it seems that there has been a very slow and gradual reduction in supply of blood to the brain, perhaps by small blood vessels becoming blocked, and it is the cumulative effects of this reduction in blood supply to the brain which cause the cognitive losses affecting memory and the ability to carry out actions of everyday living.

To be healthy and function properly, brain cells need a good supply of blood. Blood is delivered through a network of blood vessels called the vascular system. If the vascular system within the brain becomes damaged (for example, by a stroke or trauma) and blood cannot reach the brain cells, the cells will eventually die. This may lead to the onset of vascular dementia. It is now believed that vascular 'events' may also have a bearing on the development of Alzheimer's disease.

It follows that, since exercise has a beneficial effect on the cardiovascular system as a whole, it will have this effect on the part of the vascular system that supplies blood to the brain. A better supply of blood to the brain will prevent or decrease damage to the brain and the manifestation of that damage as symptoms of dementia. But vascular disease is not the whole story and in actual fact the mechanism by which physical activity improves cognition in older people (at least in those at risk of dementia) is not clear. However, the results of a significant body of research do seem to demonstrate that physical activity is key to the non-development of dementia symptoms.

J Colcombe and colleagues, in a study looking at the relationship between aerobic fitness and brain volume, observed 59 healthy but sedentary volunteers, aged 60-79 years, who were living in the community (that is, not in residential care homes). Half of the group undertook aerobic training whilst the other half participated in a toning and stretching 'control' group. Significant increases in brain volume, in both grey and white matter regions, were found after six months' trial in those who participated in the aerobic fitness training but not in those who had been taking part in the stretching and toning (non-aerobic) control group. Along with other research this study suggests that the scope of beneficial effects of aerobic exercise extend beyond just cardiovascular health, and that there is a direct effect upon brain health and volume.[2]

Danielle Laurin and colleagues, in a study coordinated through the University of Ottawa and the Division of Aging and Seniors, Health Canada, set out to explore the association between physical activity and the risk of cognitive impairment and dementia. Their research showed that, compared with no exercise, physical activity was associated with 'lower risks ... of dementia of any type'.[3] This study of a large number of people emphasised that significant trends for increased protection (from dementia) were observed with greater physical activity and this possibly protective effect was particularly noticeable in women.

One theory is that exercise has an effect on brain plasticity (see chapter 4). Carl W Cotman and Nicole C Berchtold suggested the possibility that exercise acted directly on the molecular structure of the brain itself and that beneficial effects were not simply connected with a general benefit to overall health. In an animal study using rats and mice given the opportunity (but not forced) to use an exercise wheel, Cotman and Berchtold focused on a substance called 'brain-derived neurotrophic factor' (BDNF) because it makes possible neuronal connectivity. In simple words, this factor allows neurons to connect to one another and change their connections when new skills are being learned. The researchers expected that the response to exercise would be restricted to motor sensory systems of the brain (see chapter 4) such as the cerebellum, primary cortical areas or basal ganglia. Amazingly, after several days of voluntary wheel running, they found increased levels of BDNF in the hippocampus, a part of the brain normally associated with higher cognitive function.

The hippocampus has important roles in the consolidation of information from short-term memory to long-term memory, and in spatial navigation. In Alzheimer's disease, the hippocampus is one of the first regions of the brain to suffer damage. Memory problems and disorientation appear among the first symptoms of the disease. This research indicated that exercise actually strengthens the neural structure, helping the neurons to make connections with each other.[4]

So, it appears that even a little light exercise is better than no exercise at all for our cognitive function.

The next question might be: 'Is there more improvement in cognition the more exercise you undertake?' One large-scale US study in which levels of exercise and cognitive impairment status were measured over a 10-year period was particularly interesting in this respect. The results showed not only that exercise had a beneficial affect on cognition but that the number and different types of exercise performed were inversely associated with the onset of cognitive improvement. The interesting point is that whilst exercise of any kind was found to be beneficial, the number of different types of exercise made a difference. Those engaging in four different types of exercise over a two-week period decreased their risk (of cognitive impairment) when compared with those who engaged in one type of exercise.[5] It isn't clear why different types of exercise seem to be more beneficial than just one. It is possible that taking part in a greater variety of exercise means that people get more social and cognitive stimulation in addition to the beneficial effect of exercise upon the brain.

'Exercise' in this context does not mean necessarily sweating it out in a gym. The study took account of all types of exercise, even walking and gardening, or 'yard work'.

A study involving Swedish twins investigated whether exercise earlier in life had an effect on the probability of developing dementia at a later stage. Scientists like to use twins in their research due to their 'genotypes' (that is, their genetic coding) and family environments tending to be similar (and exactly the same as far as genotype is concerned, if they are identical twins). In this research scientists were investigating whether those who exercised in mid-life (well before any signs of dementia might manifest) were less likely to become demented later in life. In this case, the researchers concluded that: 'light exercise such as gardening or walking and regular exercise involving sports were associated with reduced odds of dementia compared to hardly any exercise'.[6]

David Snowdon in his book *Aging With Grace*, an account of the well-known 'Nun Study' (see chapter 3), relates the story of a conversation with Sister Nicolette (then aged 91) in which he asks her to what she attributes her good health and longevity. She replies that she has an exercise programme which involves walking several miles a day. When asked when she started this programme, Sister Nicolette replies: 'When I was 70.' So perhaps we might query when 'mid-life' begins.

Many researchers point out that the 'exercise effect' may not be necessarily as clear cut as it appears. It could be that people who exercise more tend to lead healthier lives generally, eating a healthy diet, avoiding smoking and keeping to a moderate alcohol intake, for example. Nevertheless, the fact remains that those who exercise more have a lower risk of developing dementia in later life.

Exercise is beneficial even after memory problems have manifested themselves. There are a number of studies which link Alzheimer's disease and other dementias with a more general physical deterioration. People with dementia are more likely to show signs of under nutrition, to have a higher risk of falls (and consequent fractures) and a more rapid decline in mobility. Improving the physical condition of people with dementia may therefore extend their independent mobility and their quality of life. Even quite elderly people can improve their cardiovascular function, their ability to move muscle groups easily and without pain, their balance and their strength, with a systematic exercise programme. Improved flexibility and balance are likely to reduce the possibility of falls which may result in injury or admission to hospital. If you read chapter 9, 'If you are worried that you are developing dementia', you will realise that it is important to avoid injury and admission to hospital where at all possible. So an exercise programme is worth undertaking to improve the general health and well-being of anyone with the beginnings of dementia. Further than this, a number of studies have been carried out which look specifically at exercise-induced benefits in cognitive functioning in people with dementia.

Exercise is known to improve cardiorespiratory fitness. Building on this, a study in 2009 examined the relationship between cardiorespiratory fitness and regional brain volume in a sample of people with early Alzheimer's disease compared with non-demented 'controls' (people who were very similar in all aspects apart from not having Alzheimer's disease). In this study, those in early stage Alzheimer's with a higher level of cardiorespiratory fitness had a higher temporal lobe volume, particularly in the areas associated with executive processing. These parts of the brain are affected early in Alzheimer's disease. This seemed to apply to people carrying the **ApoE4 gene**. There have been other studies to examine whether exercise programmes will improve memory in those with early-stage dementia. A physical activity **intervention trial** was conducted in which participants who reported memory problems were encouraged to undertake 150 minutes per week of physical activity of moderate intensity. Most chose walking; a few included some light strength training as well. Participants were tested using a standard Alzheimer's disease test (**ADAS-Cog**) at the start of the trial and after six, 12 and 18 months to see if their cognitive function had improved overall and in comparison with a control 'usual care' group. The group who exercised did better in the **ADAS-Cog test** and had a better delayed recall, showing that exercise did improve cognitive function in older adults with memory problems. The improvement was apparent after six months and persisted for 12 months after discontinuation of the trial.

A 2009 study which tested the effects of a combined diet and exercise intervention in people at risk of developing Alzheimer's disease included 1800 people, 1598 of whom showed no signs of dementia at the start of the study. In consideration of the fact that elderly people are often quite inactive, this study used as its test intervention 1.3 hours per week of vigorous activity (such as aerobic dancing, jogging or playing handball), 2.4 hours of moderate exercise (such as, cycling, swimming, hiking or playing tennis), or four hours of light exercise (such as walking, playing golf, bowling, gardening), or a combination of these, to denote 'high physical activity'. In younger people this might be deemed a low amount of physical activity, but even this relatively small amount of physical activity was associated with a reduction in the risk of developing Alzheimer's disease.[9]

Patricia Heyn and colleagues conducted a 'meta-analysis' of research on exercise and dementia. A meta-analysis is a method of contrasting and combining results from different studies, in the hope of identifying patterns across study results. This paper looked at a number of **randomised trials** (studies where participants are randomly allocated to the 'intervention group' or the 'control group') with subjects (that is, participants) over 65 years of age. The authors concluded that exercise increased fitness, physical function, cognitive function, and positive behaviour in people with dementia and related cognitive impairments.[10] They also mentioned the problem of motivating people with dementia to exercise and the possible need to adjust exercise programmes to match dementia needs (see below).

Mild cognitive impairment may be an indicator of later dementia. Laura Baker conducted a study which looked at the effects of aerobic exercise on cognition in older adults with mild cognitive impairment. This was a six-month randomised controlled clinical trial, although it included only a small number (33) of participants. These participants undertook either high intensity aerobic exercise or, in the case of the control group, supervised stretching exercises. The study concluded that physical exercise had an effect on cognition, glucose metabolism and cardiac fitness. Again (as in the Lauren study), this effect was particularly noticeable in women.[11]

A randomised controlled trial by Linda Teri and colleagues, reported in a 2003 paper, investigated the effect of exercise plus a behavioural management programme given to carers of people with dementia. The exercise component of the programme included aerobic/endurance activities, strength training, balance and flexibility training, and carers were trained to instigate and supervise this exercise programme at home. In addition to the exercise programme, carers were educated about dementia and its effects and to increase physical and social activity. After three months on the programme there were definite improvements in physical functioning and, significantly, improvements in the level of depression, in those with dementia who had been randomly assigned to the exercise group compared with the 'control' group.[12] As described in chapter 1, depression often accompanies dementia and is an added difficulty, both for those diagnosed with depression and dementia and for those who are caring for them.

A further study conducted from 1993 to 2003 (so, over a long period) examined whether participation in physical activity reduced the rate of cognitive decline after accounting for participation in cognitively stimulating activities. Initially, results showed that more hours of activity were associated with a slower rate of decline in cognitive function. However, when results were adjusted to allow for the effect of cognitively stimulating activity, it was reckoned that the effect of physical activity was not significant.[13] Although this study seems at first sight to negate some other research which shows the positive effects of physical exercise, it is not as clear cut as that. Participants in the study who exercised regularly showed a slower rate of cognitive decline. What is clear is that those people who took part in regular exercise more often probably also took part in cognitively stimulating activities as well. In actual fact, physical activity is in itself cognitively stimulating and generally exercising more results also in a more full and varied social life. For example, walking might involve going to new places, meeting others during the walk and conversation in the course of the walk.

The evidence is clear even if we do not yet understand entirely why exercise makes a difference. People who exercise are less likely to develop dementia and this seems especially to apply to women. Light exercise is better than no exercise at all. It is clear too, that it is never too late to begin exercising. Those who already have signs of dementia or who have mild cognitive impairment can still obtain benefit from commencing an exercise programme. Exercise, it seems, is a wonderful prophylactic, and a treatment, and it is free. What more could you ask for?

If you or someone you care for has a memory problem, or if you or someone you care for has been diagnosed with dementia, then all the research indicates that exercise is likely to be beneficial. Some research suggests that physical exercise might be much more beneficial than so-called 'brain exercise'. As discussed, even quite moderate exercise, such as walking or gardening, will help. There is also another side to the suggestion that exercise is beneficial, as I have already suggested. Physical exercise gets you out and about, increases your number of human (and possibly animal) contacts and allows you to experience different places, scenery, weather and social situations. Research shows that plenty of social contacts, a varied social life and varied activity all help both to reduce the chance of developing dementia and to improve the prognosis if dementia is diagnosed.

If someone for whom you care has incipient memory problems or is diagnosed with dementia, then any exercise programme may be reliant on your instigation and active co-operation. In chapter 1 I explained that one of the first areas of the brain to be affected by many forms of dementia is that part which deals with the 'executive function' – the part which causes you to decide to take action. This is why many carers describe a gradual cessation of activity, even to the falling away of a previously engrossing hobby, in the years before dementia is suspected. It is also the reason why many people go to their doctor thinking that they are depressed because depression can result in a loss of interest in habitual pursuits.

****

My husband was always the chief gardener. I enjoyed everyday gardening chores but he put his heart and soul into the garden. He knew the best time for sowing and planting, spent hours caring for the lawn and was generally found out in the garden in all weathers – even rain wouldn't stop him pottering in the greenhouse or turning the compost heap. I can't remember when I started having to suggest he mowed the lawn because it was getting untidy or when exactly I started tying in climbers or pruning shrubs – all things he used to want to do. Looking back I feel that this was the beginning of what later became a general inertia and sort of lethargy – a reluctance to do anything even when prompted.

****

In such cases it may be that the carer needs to initiate and encourage any exercise programme. It is not suggested that you nag or use force and nor should you put the person with dementia into an unfamiliar situation where he/she will be under stress. So, unless you regularly visited a gym in pre-dementia days, it would be unwise to begin now. However, it is a simple thing to increase the amount of walking that takes place during everyday activities; trips to the shops or the local library, visits to friends and so on can involve some walking exercise. The requirement to give up the driving licence could be a splendid excuse to walk more. The need to walk a dog can be a very good reason to increase activity, and there is the added benefit in that most dogs will know their way home even if the person with dementia becomes confused whilst out.

Other forms of exercise, such as simple garden chores like sweeping up leaves or cutting the grass, can be done together. Taking up a new pastime may be problematic since people with dementia find it difficult to learn new things, but resuming a past activity such as bowls or swimming may be a good way to increase the potential for both exercise and increased social contacts. Dancing is a very good aerobic exercise which two people can enjoy together and which need not be presented as 'exercise', but more as an enjoyable social activity. Men of any age seem to enjoy kicking a football around and may be keen to do this with grandchildren. Remember that as a carer, if you begin to exercise more yourself you could be protecting your future too. For those whose physical impairment prevents exercise such as walking, even simple chair exercises can help. Some forms of yoga can be practised by elderly people who have a restricted range of movement, especially if props are used.[14]

There are some people with dementia who become restless and seem to have a compulsion to walk around – sometimes not stopping to sit down and rest at all during their waking hours. Others grow restless and start to walk around only at certain times of the day. Although we do not know why these people have this compulsive urge, it has been found that regular exercise planned and organised during the day can have a beneficial effect on mood and may reduce the amount of seemingly 'aimless' walking.

The balance of evidence seems to indicate that physical exercise improves or slows the decline of cognition. Whether this is proved to be a certain fact or not, it is known that there are other benefits to being as physically fit as possible. Fit and flexible people are less likely to fall and injure themselves. Regular exercise reduces the chances of developing many health problems and has a beneficial effect on mood. It is never too late to begin to increase the amount of physical exercise we undertake. After reading this chapter you might like to begin your exercise programme right away.

Key points

- Exercise is thought to benefit the cardiovascular system
- Physical exercise is associated with a lower risk of dementia of any type
- Physical exercise may also have a positive effect on brain plasticity
- The more exercise and the more different forms of exercise undertaken, the more benefit is received
- Even moderate physical exercise is of benefit
- Exercise is beneficial even for those already diagnosed with dementia
- Exercise is simple to incorporate into your daily life

References

1. NHS Choices. www.nhs.uk/Livewell
2. Colcombe SJ, et al. Aerobic exercise training increases brain volume in aging humans. *The Journals of Gerontology: Series A – Biological Sciences and Medical Sciences* 2006; 61(11): 1166-1170.
3. Laurin D, et al. Physical activity and the risk of cognitive impairment and dementia in elderly persons. *Archives of Neurology* 2001; 58(3): 498-504.
4. Cotman C W, Berchtold NC. Exercise: a behavioural intervention

to enhance brain health and plasticity. *Trends in Neoroscience* 2002; 25(6): 295-301.

5. Jedrziewski MK, et al. Exercise and cognition: results from the National Long Term Care Survey. *Alzheimer's and Dementia* 2010; 6: 448-455.

6. Andel R, et al. Physical exercise at midlife and risk of dementia three decades later: a population-based study of Swedish twins. *The Journals of Gerontology: Series A – Biological Sciences and Medical Sciences* 2008; 63(1): 62-66.

7. Honea RA, et al. Cardiorespiratory fitness and preserved medial temporal lobe volume in Alzheimer disease. *Alzheimer Disease and Associated Disorders* 2009 ; 23: 188-197.

8. Lautenschlager NT, et al. Effect of physical activity on cognitive function in older adults at risk of Alzheimer disease. *Journal of the American Medical Association* 2008; 300: 1027-1037.

9. Scarmeas N, et al. Physical activity, diet and risk of Alzheimer disease. *Journal of the American Medical Association* 2009; 302(6): 627-637.

10. Heyn P, et al. The effects of exercise training on elderly persons with cognitive impairment and dementia: a meta-analysis. *Archives of Physical Medicine and Rehabilitation* 2004; 85: 1694-1704.

11. Baker LD. Effects of aerobic exercise on mild cognitive impairment: A controlled trial. *Archives of Neurology* 2010; 67(1): 71-79. DOI: 10.1001/archneurol.2009.307.

12. Teri L, et al. Exercise plus behavioural management in patients with Alzheimer's disease: A randomized controlled trial. *Journal of the American Medical Association* 2003; 290: 2015-2022.

13. Sturman MT, et al. Physical activity, cognitive activity and cognitive decline in a biracial community population. *Archives of Neurology* 2005; 62: 1750-1754.

14. Francina S. *The New Yoga for People Over 50: a comprehensive guide for midlife and older beginners.* Florida: Health Communications; 1997.

Chapter 6

Nutrition

'You are what you eat' the saying goes, and indeed, much government health advice these days centres around what we eat, how much we eat and how we 'should' be eating. Diet related ill-health is now believed to be the leading cause of chronic disease around the world.[1] It may appear surprising then that comparatively little research has been done on the effects of diet on dementia and the risks of dementia.

Just as our bones and muscles need to be fed properly in order to function correctly, so too do our brains if they are to work at the optimal level. The physical body and the brain are both composed of body cells. The food used by the brain is glucose, of which more below.

The brain is composed of many different types of cells, but the primary functional unit is a cell called a **neuron**. All sensations, movements, thoughts, memories and feelings are the result of signals that pass through neurons. Neurons have a cell body which contains: the nucleus; **dendrites**. which extend out from the cell body like the branches of a tree and receive messages from other nerve cells; and **axons**, down which signals travel away from the cell body, to another neuron, or a muscle cell, or cells in some other organ. Some particular kinds of cells are wrapped around the axon to form an insulating sheath. This sheath can include a fatty molecule called **myelin**, which provides insulation for the axon and helps nerve signals travel faster and farther.

The place where a signal passes from the neuron to another cell is called the **synapse**. It is a minute gap; neurons do not actually quite touch each other. When the signal reaches the end of the axon of a neuron it stimulates tiny sacs in that neuron to release chemicals known as **neurotransmitters** into the synapse. The neurotransmitters cross the synapse and attach themselves to receptors on a nearby cell. If the receiving cell is also a neuron, the signal can continue the transmission to the next cell.

One neurotransmitter, acetylcholine, is classified as an 'excitatory' neurotransmitter because it generally makes cells more able to work. It governs muscle contractions and causes glands to secrete hormones. Alzheimer's disease is associated with a shortage of acetylcholine. This shortage means that signals are transmitted less easily between neurons.

The sole food of the brain is glucose (although the brain cannot store glucose), and it makes use of almost a quarter of the glucose and oxygen which the body takes in. Because the brain uses glucose as its main source of energy, it might be thought that a high level of glucose in the blood would be good, encouraging it to work better. In actual fact, fluctuations in blood glucose level, such as are caused by a diet high in carbohydrate and fructose (a type of sugar found particularly in fruit), are detrimental. The brain needs a sustained and balanced supply of glucose and this is best obtained from eating foods which cause blood glucose levels to rise more slowly and to be sustained for longer.

So, because the brain needs a sustained and balanced supply of glucose, our diet should consist of foods which will give a steady supply (see below) and not cause high peaks in blood glucose. High peaks in blood glucose level are inevitably followed by low troughs. People who are sensitive to blood sugar fluctuations (e.g. those who suffer from hypoglycaemia) know very well the feelings of edginess, irritability, shakiness and sometimes even nausea which extreme hunger can cause. People with diabetes may suffer from these symptoms if they do not control their blood sugar levels. Diabetics are taught to carry sweets or chocolate or sugar with them to avoid suffering from a 'hypo'. These sweet items will cause a swift rise in blood sugar levels, which may be beneficial in an emergency. However, it is better for everyone to eat a diet which avoids these highs and lows. We should all aim for a slow and sustained release of glucose into the blood.

Many of us were taught at school about the body's basic dietary requirements for protein, fats and carbohydrates.

Proteins: Put simply, proteins are required for bodily growth and repair of tissues, as, for example, during recovery from injury. We need proteins every day to remain healthy as our bodies cannot store them in any quantity. Proteins are made up of chains of 'amino acids'. There are eight amino acids which are essential to the body and have to be obtained from food as our bodies cannot make them. Meat, fish, eggs and dairy produce all contain the eight essential amino acids in the proportions needed by the body. Other foods, such as nuts, legumes (peas, beans and lentils) and seeds contain some of the essential amino acids and can be eaten in combination to provide the body with the right amino acid mixture. Strict vegetarians have to be careful to eat both adequate amounts and an adequate variety of protein-containing foods to ensure a sufficient supply of essential amino acids.

Fats provide energy for the growth and maintenance of body tissues and help to maintain body temperature. They also provide fat-soluble vitamins (vitamins A, D and E). A sufficient amount of fat in our diet causes us to feel full and prevents us overeating, while an excess will cause us to feel sick – it is difficult to overeat fats, unlike sugars and carbohydrates. When digested, fats break down into 'fatty acids'. To supply the fatty acids essential for proper functioning of the brain, you need to eat at least 15 grams of these each day. As well as the obvious fat on meat and in butter and cooking fats, fat is found in oily fish, milk, cheese, eggs and condiments such as mayonnaise. Some foods such as nuts have quite a high fat content, although this may not be obvious. Do not be misled by the simple (and erroneous) statement commonly read in popular literature that 'eating fat makes you fat'. When fat is digested it is oxidised by the body to provide energy for tissue activity and for the maintenance of body temperature. Deposits of fat around the vital organs of the body hold these organs in position and protect them from damage. Fat is particularly important in the structure of the brain and nervous tissue. We need a steady intake of fat for it to function properly and fats make up 60 per cent of the brain and the nerves that run every system in the body. The body needs two kinds of fat to manufacture healthy brain cells and **prostaglandins**. These fats are omega-6 (linoleic acid) and omega-3 (alpha linolenic) and are often known as **essential fatty acids**. **Cholesterol** is a fatty substance known as a 'lipid' and is vital for the normal functioning of the body. It is mainly made by the liver, but can also be found in many foods that we eat. Cholesterol is needed everywhere in the brain as an antioxidant and to manufacture the neurotransmitters, such as acetylcholine, which we have seen are the means by which nerve cells communicate.

Carbohydrates also provide energy. Most people think of things like bread and potatoes when they consider the word carbohydrates, but it is important to remember that all sugars and starches are actually carbohydrates. This includes sucrose (table sugar) and fructose, which is the sugar found in fruit. After absorption in the intestines the products of carbohydrates (sugars) are utilised to produce energy. Excess sugars are converted into fat. If insufficient carbohydrate is taken in the diet to produce the required glucose, then the body can convert fat into glucose to produce energy, and if there is not enough fat, then protein can be diverted to produce energy. It is clear that the availability of glucose is an essential for life.

Other essentials: The body also requires a supply of vitamins, minerals and trace elements to function correctly. Generally, if the diet is adequate in respect of protein, fats and carbohydrates, then a sufficient supply of vitamins, minerals and trace elements will be taken in.

Risks associated with refined carbohydrates and low fat

In order to produce the slow and sustained release of glucose mentioned previously, our diet should not be too high in carbohydrates which tend to produce a 'spike' in blood sugar levels. Every meal should contain protein, fat and a limited amount of carbohydrate, and meals should be eaten at regular intervals. If they are properly balanced and eaten regularly, then additional snacks should not be necessary or even desired. This doesn't mean that you should not treat yourself to the odd slice of cake with your afternoon tea. It means that if you actually need that slice of cake in order to last out until the next meal, then either your diet is not properly balanced or your meals are too far apart from each other.

Standard current dietary advice is based around what is considered to be 'good' for the health of our heart and cardiac system. Broadly, the advice is to base our diet around carbohydrates, to reduce our intake of fats, increase our intake of fruit and vegetables and to keep cholesterol levels low. Whilst this diet is popularly considered to be a 'healthy heart diet' for those in mid-life, some specific research shows that in adopting this way of eating we are no longer giving our brain the optimum diet. As explained above, in order to work properly the brain needs dietary fat, cholesterol and a steady intake of glucose.

What is becoming clear from research is that there is a definite link between excess dietary carbohydrates (particularly refined carbohydrates and, above all, the sugar called fructose) along with a deficiency in dietary fats and cholesterol which may lead to the development of Alzheimer's disease.

One paper, published in the *Journal of Neurochemistry* in 2008, points out that in trials, a reduced carbohydrate intake prevented Alzheimer's disease-type **amyloidosis** (a condition where proteins are abnormally deposited in organs or tissues and cause harm). This paper mentions the term 'metabolic syndrome' which is used to describe a group of risk factors that occur together and are thought to increase the risk for coronary artery disease, stroke and type 2 diabetes. The suggestion is that this syndrome also increases the risk for Alzheimer's disease and the syndrome is linked to high calorie intake and diets high in sugar and refined flour. The authors recommend that those at risk of Alzheimer's disease eat whole and unrefined foods with natural fats, especially fish, nuts and seeds, olives and olive oil, and reduce the intake of foods that disrupt insulin and the blood sugar balance.[2]

A 2011 paper published in the *European Journal of Internal Medicine* points out that the cerebrospinal fluid in the brains of people with Alzheimer's disease is deficient in fats and cholesterol and suggests that Alzheimer's disease may be caused by a deficiency in the supply chain of cholesterol, fats and antioxidants to the brain. This paper suggests that a diet high in high-glycaemic carbohydrates (especially fructose) and low in cholesterol and fats begins the process that leads to neuronal failure. The authors propose that dietary modifications resulting in fewer highly processed carbohydrates and more fats and cholesterol are a protective measure against Alzheimer's disease. We have seen that neurons are involved in the transmission of signals in the brain. **Astrocytes** are the cells that supply cholesterol and fats to the neurons. It is believed that excess exposure to glucose and to oxidising agents can lead to damage in the astrocytes. This, say the authors of the paper, leads to defects in the transmission of neural signals.[3]

Recent animal-based research has suggested that cutting calories overall may halt or even reverse the symptoms of Alzheimer's disease. Published in the *Journal of Alzheimer's Disease*, this study involved a team of researchers from the Mount Sinai School of Medicine in New York City maintaining a group of squirrel monkeys on either calorie-restrictive or normal diets throughout their lifespan. Compared to those on a normal diet, the monkeys that were fed the reduced-calorie diet were less likely to have Alzheimer's disease-type changes in their brain.[4]

The reduced-calorie diet was also associated with increased longevity of a protein known as SIRT1, which influences a variety of functions, including age-related diseases. The significance of this research is reflected in the further studies around ketones (see below).

However, when considering a reduced-calorie diet it is also important to remember that many elderly people may be in a poor nutritional state due to increasing frailty, lack of exposure to sunlight and inability to shop for food and prepare meals because of cognitive impairment or physical disability. If someone is already suffering from under-nutrition it would be quite inappropriate to suggest a reduction in calories. Instead, action to enrich the diet should be taken in accordance with the suggestions given at the end of this chapter.

Research has already indicated a clear link between Alzheimer's disease and diabetes (see chapter 8 on physical disease). A diet high in processed carbohydrates like white bread, breakfast cereals and fruit juices, particularly if this diet is also low in fats, results in a rapid rise in blood glucose levels after meals. Over time it is believed that this may lead to insulin resistance and diabetes.

One of the most interesting links between nutrition and the risk of dementia was the subject of a piece of research which showed a link between the nutritional status of mothers in pregnancy and the development of dementia in their children in later life. At the end of World War II a severe famine occurred in cities in the western part of the Netherlands. At one stage the rations were as low as 400 calories per day. This study found that in late middle life (age 56-59 years) people exposed to famine during the early stage of gestation performed worse than expected on selective attention tasks.[5]

Eating a well-balanced diet will give a controlled release of glucose, ensure we have the nutrients we need to stay healthy and help to protect against dementia. But what truly is a well-balanced diet? Research information indicates that not all current 'accepted' advice about low-fat/high-carbohydrate diets and restricted cholesterol should necessarily apply to older people wishing to protect themselves against dementia. It appears that simple dietary modification towards fewer highly processed carbohydrates and relatively more fats and cholesterol is likely to be a protective measure against Alzheimer's disease.

Omega-6 and omega-3

As was mentioned earlier in this chapter, omega-6 and omega-3 are often known as essential fatty acids as they must be obtained from our food; we cannot make them ourselves. There are three types of omega-3: alpha-linolenic acid (ALA), eicosapentaenoic acid (EPA) and docosahexaenoic acid (DHA). ALA is thought to help reduce heart disease and EPA and DHA help maintain the tissues of the eye and brain.

Omega-6 has two types: linoleic acid (LA) and arachidonic acid (AA). These are the prime structural components of brain cell membranes and are also an important part of the enzymes within cell membranes that allow the transport of valuable nutrients in and out of the cells.

Omega-6 is found in a variety of foods, including meat and animal products such as eggs, and it is believed that a shortage of this fat is rare in most western diets. Omega-3 is found generally in oily fish as well as in some oils, nuts and seeds. Most current advice centres around the suggestion that we increase our intake of omega-3 in order to balance our intake of omega-6. However, the simple fact is that there is very little consensus among nutritionists about how much omega-3 and omega-6 oils are needed in total for optimum health and about the ideal ratio between the two. While there is a theory that omega-3 fatty acids are better for our health than omega-6 fatty acids, this is not necessarily supported by the latest evidence.

As far as there is any consensus, it seems to centre on the suggestion that for the health of our hearts and our brains we should all be eating more oily fish. A research paper looking at fish consumption and cognitive function in people without dementia showed that: 'there were significant positive associations between reported fish consumption and the CVLT (Californian Verbal Learning Test) scores.' It concluded: 'we have demonstrated a positive association between reported fish consumption and cognitive function in a large sample of healthy older people in the UK.'[6]

The usual recommendation is two servings of oily fish per week. The word 'oily' seems to put many people off, but in fact this term includes a number of different species which makes it easier to include these in the diet: mackerel, herring, salmon, whitebait, sardines, trout, pilchards, kippers, eels, fresh tuna, anchovies, swordfish and sprats. Tinned tuna is not included in this list because the canning process is thought to negate the omega-3 content. However, high-quality brands canned in water rather than oil can in fact contain significant amounts. You need to read the label.

Vegetarians can get omega-3 from flax-seed, hemp-seed, nuts and (if eaten) eggs. Given such a comprehensive list you may begin to think that increasing our omega-3 intake is not really very difficult.

Ketones

An interesting piece of information and anecdotal evidence has come from the USA. A Florida doctor, Dr Mary Newport, who is married to someone who has dementia, read some information about coconut oil and begun dosing her husband with this. She claims that he has shown a remarkable improvement on this regime and has submitted some of his test results to bear out his recovery.[7] The improvements in her husband's cognition have not all been maintained and this type of initial promise followed by a disappointing follow-up is common to many of the 'exciting break-though' research headlines in the popular press. No serious research has been done on the benefits of coconut oil in the UK, but the theoretical reasoning behind this supplement is borne out by nutritional knowledge which indicates that the brain can use ketones for nourishment when glucose is unavailable. The first placebo-controlled trial of coconut oil is just beginning in Florida USA and many will await the results with interest.

Research has been done which involves using mice to test the effect of a high-fat/low-carbohydrate diet. The conclusion of this research states: 'Here we demonstrate that a diet rich in saturated fats and low in carbohydrates can actually reduce levels of Abeta [amyloid beta]. Therefore, dietary strategies aimed at reducing Abeta [amyloid beta] levels should take into account interactions of dietary components and the metabolic outcomes, in particular, levels of carbohydrates, total calories, and presence of ketone bodies, should be considered.'[8] Of course it needs to be remembered that not all animal-based research translates into benefits in humans.

A US-based, 90-day, **randomised, double-blind, placebo-controlled, parallel-group study** which involved giving people with early to moderate Alzheimer's disease (AD) an oral ketogenic compound, resulted in significant differences in **ADAS-Cog** scores between those taking the compound and the placebo group. The authors concluded: 'Therefore, chronic induction of ketosis may offer a novel strategy for AD that can be used with current therapies'.[9]

Supplements

There have been a number of trials of various dietary supplements (other than coconut oil) to test whether they are effective in preventing dementia and whether these supplements improve symptoms in those who already have dementia. A problem with such trials is the fact that any dietary supplementation takes time to show its effects. This means any trials have to be carried out over a long period of time. In addition, trials usually have to be carried out using specific pre-packaged supplements – perhaps in pill form - which make it easy for participants to take part. Trying to ensure that participants in a trial eat particular foods in sufficient quantities is much more difficult. Below is a summary of the current status of some of the trials.

B vitamins

Significant research has been carried out around B vitamins, particularly folic acid. It has been noted that a rise in blood levels of a particular amino acid called homocysteine is associated with an increased risk of Alzheimer's disease and vascular dementia as well as stroke and heart disease. At this present time it is still not clear whether raised homocysteine levels are a pointer to an increased risk of dementia and heart disease (including stroke) or whether raised levels are *caused* by heart disease and dementia. Supplements of folic acid (also called vitamin B9) can be shown to lower the levels of homocysteine in the blood and for a while this line of research appeared very exciting. However, trials have shown that even when homocysteine levels are reduced, this does not restore cognitive function in those people with early stage dementia, nor does it appear to improve the prognosis for those with cardiac problems. Further research into the efficacy of vitamin B is ongoing, and this still looks like a promising area. It needs to be noted that the levels of B vitamins used in the trials were much higher than can usually be obtained in our diets or by taking supplements. Therefore no causal effect of (for example) a low level of B vitamins in those who develop dementia is suggested at this stage.

Vitamin D

Some research has been carried out into the connection between low levels of vitamin D and dementia. Levels of this vitamin are often low in older people and are also lower in the general population than a generation ago. The reason seems to be that the main source of vitamin D for the body is from the action of sunlight on the skin. Many older people, especially those living in residential care homes, may not go out into the sun very much. In addition a great deal of publicity has been given to the connection between skin cancer and sunlight-damage to the skin, and the use of sunscreen cream is much higher than it used to be. The *American Journal of Alzheimer's Disease and Other Dementias* reported in a paper published in 1997 that: 'Patients with Alzheimer's disease in particular have a high prevalence of vitamin D deficiency, which is also associated with low mood and impaired cognitive performance in older people.' The authors noted that: 'Vitamin D clearly has a beneficial role in AD [Alzheimer's disease] and improves cognitive function in some patients with AD.'[10]

Given that current advice is to apply high-factor sunscreen and to avoid direct sunlight in the middle of the day (the time when the action of sun on the skin is most effective at producing vitamin D) this research finding is clearly very interesting, if, perhaps, controversial.

Vitamin E

Vitamin E is an 'antioxidant' – that is, a substance that scientists believe may protect brain cells and other body tissues from certain kinds of chemical wear and tear. A 1997 study showed that high doses of vitamin E delayed loss of ability to carry out daily activities and placement in residential care by several months.[11] However, since the study was carried out, scientists have found evidence in other studies that high-dose vitamin E may slightly increase the risk of death, especially for those with coronary artery disease. Vitamin E in high doses can interact with other medications, including those prescribed to keep blood from clotting or to lower cholesterol. Therefore, vitamin E supplements should be taken with caution and only after checking with your doctor.

Ginkgo biloba

Ginkgo biloba is a herbal supplement which has a reputation for improving learning and memory. Initial research published in 2002 seemed to show promise for application of its properties to help those diagnosed with dementia.[12] This fitted with the reputation of the herb, and its use by herbalists for the improvement of memory in students studying for examinations. However, in a later study published in the *Journal of the American Medical Association*, 240 milligrams per day was found to be ineffective in reducing the development of dementia in general, and Alzheimer's disease in particular, in older people. This study, known as the 'GEM' (Ginkgo Evaluation of Memory) study, led by Steven T. DeKosky, MD, is the largest clinical trial ever to evaluate ginkgo's effect on the occurrence of dementia.[13]

Some medical herbalists have claimed that the dose used was insufficient to achieve effective improvement. The fact is that, unfortunately, clinical trials have not shown consistently that ginkgo helps to prevent cognitive loss in normal elderly subjects, or to improve cognitive function in patients already diagnosed with Alzheimer's disease. Doctors are therefore not convinced of any benefit from this supplement.

Aluminium

Aluminium is not regarded as a food supplement but I am discussing its possible link with dementia here because it can be absorbed by the body via the food chain.

As was described in chapter 1, people with Alzheimer's disease have typical changes in brain organisation that are called 'neurofibrillary tangles'. Beginning in the 1960s, various studies have found high concentrations of aluminium at autopsy in the brains of people suffering from Alzheimer's disease – and almost always in the characteristic **neurofibrillary tangles** in the brain. However, other studies have found no difference between the **overall** amount of aluminium in the brains of people with Alzheimer's and the amount in normal brains. It seems the neurofibrillary tangles are very 'sticky' and absorb aluminium.

When patients with chronic kidney failure began to be routinely treated with a new technique called 'dialysis', this technique used hundreds of litres of water each day to purify the blood. Unfortunately, the aluminium naturally present in the water entered the blood, and couldn't be removed – because the kidneys of those with kidney failure were not working. As the blood levels of aluminium soared to thousands of times higher than normal, the patients became confused and demented. We now know that this 'dialysis encephalopathy' can be rectified by removing any aluminium from the water used for dialysis.

Although aluminium seemed to be implicated as a cause of

dementia, the findings described above have led to the conclusion that it is not the main causal factor in Alzheimer's disease, or other forms of dementia. None of the evidence so far has proved that aluminium contributes to the degenerative changes which cause Alzheimer's disease and the risk from increased exposure is considered to be small in general terms. However, there is little doubt that aluminium is neurotoxic (poisonous to brain cells) and excessive intake should be avoided. If you are worried about the risk, you can avoid cooking acidic foods in aluminium pans, reduce your intake of antacids (which usually contain aluminium), avoid the food additive E173 and filter your drinking water.

Conclusions

If you have been diagnosed with dementia, or if you are caring for someone with this diagnosis, you can make useful changes to the diet. You can switch to using full-fat milk and include plenty of eggs, cheese and butter in the diet. You can also include oily fish several times per week. (Some people prefer a fish-oil supplement.) You can ensure that you or the person you care for eats more unprocessed foods (for example, brown rice and wholemeal bread) and reduces consumption of processed carbohydrates and **hydrogenated fat**.

Although research so far has not shown food supplements to be the magic answer to dementia, there is no reason why you should not include supplements in the diet provided you follow recommended guidelines. So, for example, if you want to include a multi-vitamin or coconut oil or ginkgo biloba in the diet, this is unlikely to be harmful.

Above all, keep the consumption of refined sugar to a minimum. People with dementia often seem to crave sweet things (this may be connected with the brain's loss of ability to process glucose efficiently), including alcohol. Alcohol consumption needs to be supervised, if only for the simple reason that someone with dementia may forget how much alcohol they have consumed and may unwittingly drink to excess. It should also be remembered that, where the action of the brain is already impaired, alcoholic drinks will be likely to make the brain processes even slower.

In some people with dementia, the sense of taste changes so that appetite may decrease. Where people with dementia live alone, their diet is often poor. They may forget to eat regularly; they may lose the skills of cooking and revert to eating easily prepared food such as biscuits and cake. Agency helpers employed to prepare meals may (due to a shortage of time) deliver only cook-chill foods of limited nutritive content. Well-meaning family members may also see such meals as useful due to the fact that they can be quickly prepared and need little cooking skill. Often relatives and carers fall back on fortified meal replacement drinks which are frequently rich in sugar. Of course, any food is better than none and all these options help to prevent starvation. However, someone suffering from a progressive and terminal disease (which is what dementia is) deserves the best nutrition available.

People in the later stages of dementia often lose weight so it is then even more important to ensure that whatever they eat is nutrient rich. This is the reason for the advice above on giving full fat milk, plenty of eggs and cheese. If weight loss is significant, food can be fortified and advice on the best way to manage this can be obtained from the Community Mental Health Team or a dementia support worker.

Key points

- Our bodies need a balance of protein, fat and carbohydrate
- Fats and cholesterol are essential for the brain to function
- Eating oily fish is considered to be protective against dementia
- Some research suggests that cutting calories from carbohydrates may help prevent dementia
- Some vitamins and supplements may help but evidence for this is not robust
- If you have dementia you should eat a 'nutrient rich' diet

References

1. WHO Global status report on non-communicable disease 2010.2011. www.who.int/nmh/publications/ncd_report_full_en.pdf
2. Pasinetti GM, Eberstein JA. Metabolic syndrome and the role of dietary lifestyles in Alzheimer's disease. *Journal of Neurochemistry* 2008; 106: 1503-1514.
3. Seneff S, et al. Nutrition and Alzheimer's disease: The detrimental role of a high carbohydrate diet. *European Journal of Internal Medicine* 2011; DOI: 10.1016/j.jim.2010.12.017
4. Quin W, et al. Calorie restriction attenuates Alzheimer's disease type brain amyloidosis in Squirrel monkeys (Saimiri sciureus). *Journal of Alzheimer's Disease* 2006; 10(4): 417-422.
5. deRooij SR, et al. Prenatal undernutrition and cognitive function in late adulthood. *Proceedings of the National Academy of Sciences* 2010; 107(39): 16881-16886.
6. Dangour AD, et al. Fish consumption and cognitive function among

older people in the UK: Baseline Data from the OPAL Study. *Journal of Nutrition Health and Aging* 2009; 13: 198-202.

7. Newport M. *Alzheimer's: What if there was a cure?* Basic Health Publications: 2011.

8. van der Auwera I, Wera S, van Leuven F, Henderson ST. A ketogenic diet reduces amyloid beta 40 and 42 in a mouse model of Alzheimer's disease. *Nutrition & Metabolism* 2005; 2: 28. DOI:10.1186/1743-7075-2-28

9. Henderson ST, et al. Study of the ketogenic agent AC-1202 in mild to moderate Alzheimer's disease: a randomised, double- blind placebo controlled trial. Bio-med Central open access article. *Nutrition & Metabolism* 2009; 6: 31. DOI:10.1186/1743-7075-6-31

10. Lu'o'ng KVQ, Nguyen LTH. The beneficial role of vitamin D in Alzheimer's disease. *American Journal of Alzheimer's Disease and Other Dementias* 2011; 26(7): 511-520. DOI: 10.1177/1533317511429321

11. Sano M, et al. A controlled trial of selegiline, alpha-tocopherol, or both as treatment for Alzheimer's disease. The Alzheimer's Disease Cooperative Study. *New England Journal of Medicine* 1997; 336(17): 1216-1222.

12. Le Bars PL, et al. Influence of the severity of cognitive impairment on the effect of the ginkgo biloba extract EGb 761® in Alzheimer's disease. *Neuropsychobiology* 2002; 45(1): 19–26. DOI: 10.1159/000048668

13. DeKosky ST, et al. Ginkgo biloba for prevention of dementia. A randomized controlled trial. *Journal of the American Medical Association* 2008; 300(19): 2253-2262.

Chapter 7

Trauma

This chapter looks at possible connections between trauma and dementia. Trauma can be physical, due to a blow to the head or damage to the body from, for example, a traffic accident. Alternatively, it may be of a psychological nature, caused by repeated distress in the past, the stress and horror of being involved in something like a bomb incident, or what used to be known as 'battle fatigue' and is now frequently classed as 'post-traumatic stress'.

Head injury

We know that trauma to the head can result in dementia either immediately or many years after the original event. In particular, we know that repeated trauma to the head, as is experienced for example by boxers, can result in dementia in later life. **Dementia pugilistica** is the neurodegenerative disease that may affect amateur or professional boxers and also athletes in other sports who suffer concussions or near concussions. The symptoms and signs of dementia pugilistica develop progressively over a long (apparently latent) period of sometimes several decades. In people with this condition, the **neurofibrillary tangles** associated with Alzheimer's disease are observed in very high densities in the brain. However, in Alzheimer's disease, these tangles have been found to display different distribution patterns from those in dementia pugilistica cases. In dementia pugilistica, they were found to be concentrated in the superficial layers of the brain – the 'neocortex' – whereas in Alzheimer's disease they predominated in the deep layers.[1]

Dementia pugilisitca is thought to affect around 15-20 per cent of professional boxers. It is caused by repeated concussive blows and blows that are below the threshold of force necessary to cause concussion, or a mixture of the two. Soccer players are also prone to develop a similar condition due to the constant 'heading' of heavy leather footballs. The replacement of leather balls with lighter synthetic materials has now made such a possibility less likely.

Trauma to the head resulting from injury in an accident can also result in dementia. Sometimes this occurs immediately following the accident, in which case it is clear that the trauma was responsible for the dementia. However, sometimes there appears to be a complete recovery from the head trauma, but dementia develops a long time later – perhaps many years later. In this case, it is not always so clear that the head injury was the cause.

There is a body of research examining a link between head injury and dementia. As an example, Plassman and colleagues published a paper investigating head injury in early adulthood and the later risk of dementia. The results showed that moderate and severe head injuries are linked to the development of Alzheimer's disease, and dementia in general, although there was little evidence to show that minor head injury had any effect on a later risk of dementia.[2] Since this research was based on historical records, the authors pointed out that they could not exclude the possibility that other factors were involved in the later development of dementia.

A number of studies have indicated the importance of the connection between severe head injury and the possibility of accelerated neurodegenerative processes affecting the **beta amyloid plaques** which are believed to be the root cause of dementia of the Alzheimer's type.[3,4,5] This body of research indicates that the head injury itself does not cause dementia at the time but that the injury seems to precipitate a degenerative process that can result in dementia at a later date. This might tie in with the current thinking that a neurological 'event' is required to trigger dementia even in the presence of the plaques and tangles generally associated with Alzheimer's disease. A piece of research by Richard Mayeux and colleagues examined the connections between traumatic head injury and a **gene** called 'apolipoprotein-epsilon 4' (**ApoE4**). People who had a history of traumatic head injury and carried the gene ApoE4 had a 10-fold increased risk of developing Alzheimer's disease. In this study, no increased risk of dementia was found due to head injury in those who did not carry the gene ApoE4. This suggests that head injury may increase the risk of Alzheimer's disease, but only through a synergistic relationship with ApoE4.[6]

These findings might help to explain why not everyone who receives a moderate to severe head injury goes on to develop dementia, and most researchers are careful to point out that there are a number of indications for further research. If, for example, it could be proved that a traumatic brain injury accelerated the neurodegenerative processes underlying Alzheimer's disease, then interventions designed to block or reverse these processes could potentially be given to anyone with a head injury.

What might seem obvious is that precautions to protect oneself from head injury are extremely important. The cyclist's or climber's helmet is not just to prevent immediate death or injury, but may have greater long-term benefits than at first imagined.

Other forms of physical trauma

Cerebrovascular damage

Damage to blood vessels in the brain, or 'cerebrovascular damage', is a common biological cause of dementia. This includes strokes and/or narrowing of the blood vessels supplying the brain. Localised areas of the brain are destroyed (commonly called 'infarcts') from not getting enough blood supply.

Many of the same factors that cause heart disease also cause cerebrovascular disease. The type of dementia that results from cerebrovascular disease is known as **vascular dementia**. However, more and more doctors are coming to believe that the dividing line between Alzheimer's disease and vascular dementia is less clear cut than was formerly thought to be the case. There is a growing belief that a vascular event is required to cause dementia even if the plaques and tangles that indicate Alzheimer's disease are present (see chapter 2, About dementia).

In someone who has been diagnosed with dementia, it is known that any injury to any part of the body, or any infection, can result in a worsening of the symptoms. This degeneration may be temporary or permanent.[7, 8]

Delirium following anaesthetic

Following an operation under general anaesthetic, some people develop a severe (and temporary) form of confusion, often termed 'post-operative delirium'. This confusion is not dementia as such, but it is known that people who suffer from it are more likely to suffer from dementia at a later date.[9, 10] Some doctors believe that anaesthesia (possibly in combination with the pain and trauma of the operation itself) may cause a form of dementia to develop subsequent to the operation itself. Many people complain that after major surgery they are more easily tired, unable to concentrate and have memory problems and other cognitive difficulties. It is known that anaesthetic drugs linger in the body for some time. The body eliminates drugs (including anaesthetic drugs) by metabolism and excretion. It is possible that residual low concentrations may exert effects for longer than is generally believed, but while these residual effects may linger, eventually they *should* disappear completely.

However, the fact is that many relatives of people with dementia date the appearance of the symptoms from a major operation or procedure in which an anaesthetic was used. This has generally been explained away by the medical profession as coincidence or as the result of the stay in hospital increasing confusion until it becomes apparent to close relatives. It is possible that this is the case. There is no proof that an ordinary medical procedure can actually cause dementia.

Of course, no one would wish to refuse an essential operative procedure because of possible short-term anaesthetic effects. It does, however, make sense that, if you are having an elective procedure (that is, where you have notice of the date of the operation), you ensure that you are in as good a state of general health as possible when you are admitted to hospital, that the medical staff have correct information about your state of health and that you discuss any possible after effects with your surgeon beforehand. You can also make sure that those nearest to you understand about the effects of anaesthesia so that they will not be taken aback should you appear distracted or forgetful in the days following the procedure.

Where someone has actually been diagnosed with dementia, then the benefit or otherwise of any elective procedure should be considered carefully in the light of the known possibility that an operation and a stay in hospital may increase any confusion, perhaps permanently. Constant pain can also increase confusion and anxiety. The pros and cons of any medical procedure should be discussed carefully with a doctor who understands dementia.

Psychological trauma

Relatives of those with dementia frequently ask whether past psychological trauma can be the cause of current dementia. Some studies have been done on this subject. A small study published in 2010 investigated the relationship between childhood exposure to trauma and cognitive function in 47 adults. This study concluded that physical neglect and emotional abuse in childhood might be associated with memory deficits in adulthood.[11] The authors stated: 'Our observations lend support for the hypothesis that exposure to childhood trauma, especially emotional abuse and physical neglect, leads to problems in long-term and working memory in adulthood.'

Such studies are, however, not easy to conduct. People who have dementia may not be able to give an accurate history of past traumatic events. Although memories of the distant past are often well remembered, people with dementia may have difficulty in articulating them and their carers may not know all the facts, particularly if the trauma happened in childhood.

Stress

Stress is not in itself a bad thing, but too much stress of a kind which is associated with helplessness (that is, with being unable to affect the cause of the stress) is believed to be harmful to physical health. When we experience a stressful situation, the human body naturally responds physically in a rapid, automatic process commonly known as the 'fight-or-flight' reaction, or the 'stress response'. In this response, the nervous system responds to a stressful stimulus by releasing a flood of stress hormones, including adrenaline and cortisol. These hormones rouse the body for emergency action. As a result, the heart beats faster, muscles tighten, blood pressure rises, breath quickens, and senses become sharper. These physical changes increase the body's strength and stamina, speed reaction time, and enhance focus – preparing the person experiencing stress either to fight or to flee from the danger at hand. So far, so good. Where stress is thought to affect health is when the situation prevents the body from either fighting or fleeing. For example, if your boss is in a bad mood and takes his temper out on you, the employee, you are prevented by the social situation from either shouting at him/her, expressing your rage by perhaps hitting him or her, or escaping from the situation by running away. If you are a carer and the person you are caring for tries your temper too hard, you are prevented by decency and convention from getting angry and shouting or hitting them or perhaps, because of safety concerns, from walking out of the house and leaving them alone.

Work-related stress is often thought to be particularly bad for health because it causes a feeling of disempowerment, particularly in harsh financial climates when leaving and finding another job may not be a viable option. In addition to this difficulty, stress at work can be regular and continuous. Work plays a major part in the lives of most people. It improves our confidence or undermines it. Work gives us a reason to love life or a reason to hate it. Much research has been done on the effect of work-related stress on health, and some of this has concentrated on the relationship between work-related stress and the possibility of an increased risk of dementia.

A 2012 paper relates research by Hui-Xin Wang and colleagues which tests the hypothesis that high job stress during working life might lead to an increased risk of dementia in later life. The research, conducted in Sweden, looked at stress at work connected with both demands of the job and control over the job. The researchers' findings indicated that lifelong stress at work, characterised by a low level of control over the job, in combination with either high or low job demands, might increase the risk of developing dementia in later life.[12]

Several animal studies have indicated a link between chronic stress and dementia, and the Alzheimer's Society is currently conducting research into this connection.[13, 14]

Post-traumatic stress

Post-traumatic stress disorder (PTSD) has been more extensively researched. A study of over 181,000 US veterans (who have a high incidence of this disorder), published in 2010, showed that 10.6 per cent who suffered from PTSD developed dementia compared with 6.6 per cent of those who had not suffered from PTSD. When adjustments had been made to exclude other complicating factors, such as head injury, the results indicated a two-fold higher risk of developing dementia.[15] The researchers tried to identify reasons why those who suffered from PTSD might be more prone to developing dementia. One possibility suggested was that chronic stress might damage the hippocampus (the area of the brain first affected in most dementias) and the authors found some corroborating evidence for this, but other possibilities were also cited. There is also the possibility that PTSD is a direct cause of dementia or that the two conditions occur together. PTSD symptoms often get worse as people develop dementia.

Most of the subjects of the PTSD research were male. Another piece of research has looked at the relationship between psychological stress in mid-life and the later incidence of dementia in a sample of women. This was a very long study, which had a 35-year follow-up period, so the results are very interesting. (Short studies can tend to 'skew' results.) Women who reported stress on more than one occasion were more likely to develop dementia. The more frequently stress was reported (therefore indicating a more prolonged period of stress), the more likely the women were to develop dementia. Frequent constant stress between the ages of 38 and 60 years of age was associated with the development of Alzheimer's disease in later life. Interestingly, this association was recorded for both early-onset and later-onset dementia.[16]

The authors stated that it was not always possible to identify the number of each type of dementia that developed in the people taking part in the trial. The authors also pointed out the possibility that the stress might be a predictor of future dementia rather than a cause. In this respect, we need to remember that changes in the brain may appear many years before signs of dementia are obvious (see chapter 8 on physical and mental health, for further discussion of stress and mental health and dementia).

It is very common for a person with dementia to seem to become fixated on a past traumatic event, to appear to be 'reliving' the event and to speak of it often and with fear. Naturally this makes carers question whether the stress of that traumatic event caused the dementia. It is very difficult to ascertain whether this might be so. Sometimes carers suggest that therapy for the post-traumatic stress might relieve the dementia or effect a 'cure'. However, the very nature of dementia means that the mind will begin to revert to the more distant past. With most forms of dementia, recent memories are lost first whilst older memories may remain crystal clear. This is the reason that some people with dementia begin to ask to return 'home' even though they have lived in the same house for a number of years. Their memories of home are now of an earlier home, perhaps the house they lived in when they were first married, or their childhood home. This memory reversion also explains why some people with dementia periodically start to get restless and worry that they have to 'pick up the children from school', or perhaps tell you that their mother will be worrying about them even though their mother has been dead for many years. To such people the past memories are much clearer than recent events. This means that a traumatic childhood event such as running down the garden to the air raid shelter whilst bombs were dropping, or searching for their father when they had become lost in the park, is vivid and real, and may even seem to be taking place now.

When this happens it is natural that relatives will start to think that the traumatic event is the cause of the dementia. Another common idea is that with some psychiatric treatment, or with therapy from a psychologist, these vivid and upsetting memories can be laid to rest so that, even if the dementia cannot be cured, the distress can be mitigated. Unfortunately this kind of medical therapy requires some insight on the part of the patient and an ability to work through the distress and come to terms with it. This is no longer possible for someone with dementia. However, it is sometimes possible for carers to 'work through' these feelings with the person who has dementia in another way.

There is a tendency on the part of care staff, and some health professionals, to suggest that the best option with this kind of distress is to distract the person with dementia, and indeed, usually people with dementia are easily distracted. However, such diversion is self-defeating. Usually the person with dementia, after being distracted, reverts back to his/her original worry, perhaps even in a heightened way. A more workable solution is for the carer to acknowledge the feelings of the person with dementia whilst not allowing them to believe that the memories they are living through are real at the moment. It is worth remembering that even when memories are lost or the ability to follow a logical sequence has gone, the feelings and emotions of someone with dementia remain intact, and it is these feelings and emotions that people with dementia are experiencing when they are distressed. The carer might say, for example:

'You must miss your mother.'

'I expect you felt very frightened.'

'It must have been terrifying hearing the bombs.'

Often this leads the person with dementia to follow up, even if only in a very small way. A conversation of sorts may develop out of this kind of acknowledgement of feelings, and after some discussion it may be that the fear and disturbance can be laid to rest. If this does not happen, it is still better to acknowledge the feelings that have arisen whilst at the same time providing reassurance.

'It must have been frightening hearing the bombs, but there aren't any bombs now. It's all quiet.'

'I expect you were very frightened when you got lost, but luckily your father found you quickly. You are safe now.'

Peter Whitehouse in his book *The Myth of Alzheimer's* discusses this form of therapy, which is often called 'validation therapy' and is based on the idea of validating the world which the person with dementia seems to be inhabiting instead of trying to re-orient them to what we see as reality. He suggests that validation therapy helps 'elders resolve their unfinished life issues, reducing stress and enhancing dignity and quality of life.'[17] Not all dementia 'experts' agree with the theory of validation, however.

****

My father developed what seemed to be an illogical fear of the war memorial which we passed every day on our normal walk. Usually I tried to hurry him past and distract his attention. One day though when he stopped by the memorial and became agitated, I said, 'It is very sad to think of those young men who died.' To my surprise he answered, 'Yes, they were all in the Air Force with me you know.' And I realised that he was thinking about his time during the war and feeling sad about his mates who had been killed. He was a bit muddled because of course the names on the memorial were not those with whom he had served, but after that he was less upset on our walk and sometimes spontaneously said as we passed the memorial something to the effect that he was glad the war was over now.

****

Conclusions

Physical trauma in the form of head injury and its connection with dementia has been well documented and researched. Other serious illnesses and major surgical procedures may appear to onlookers to be a causative factor in dementia, but this cannot be proven. There is also some evidence that suggests that chronic stress may play a part in dementia risk. The evidence for any effect by psychological factors is less clear, but many relatives and carers suggest that this may have played a vital part in causing dementia. It is also well known that those with dementia often relive past stressful or frightening moments of their lives.

Key points

- Dementia can occur as a result of head injury
- Repeated head injury carries a higher risk of dementia
- Cerebrovascular damage can result in dementia
- People who suffer from delirium following general anaesthetic are more likely to develop dementia
- Stress and psychological trauma in early or mid-life may be factors in dementia risk
- Those who experience post-traumatic stress disorder are at a higher risk of developing dementia
- Someone who has dementia may develop worse symptoms when stressed
- People with dementia can sometimes appear to be reliving stressful times from the past
- 'Validation' of this distress can be helpful but remains controversial

References

1. Hof PR, et al. Differential distribution of neurofibrillary tangles in the cerebral cortex of dementia pugilistica and Alzheimer's disease cases. *Acta Neuropathologica* 1992; 85(1):23-30. DOI: 10.1007/BF00304630.

2. Plassman BL, Havlik RJ, Steffens DC, et al. Documented head injury in early adulthood and the risk of Alzheimer's disease and other dementias. *Neurology* 2000; 55(8): 1158-1166.

3. Roberts GW, Gentleman SM, Lynch A, et al. Beta amyloid protein deposition in the brain after severe head injury: implications for the pathogenesis of Alzheimer's disease. *Journal of Neurology Neurosurgery and Psychiatry* 1994; 57(4): 419-425.

4. Smith DH, Chen X-H, Iwata A, Graham DI. Amyloid Beta accumulation in axons after traumatic brain injury in humans. *Journal of Neurosurgery* 2003; 98(5): 1072-1077.

5. Nicoll JA, Roberts GW, Graham DI. Apolipoprotein E epsilon4 allele is associated with deposition of amyloid beta-protein following head injury. *Nature Medicine* 1995; 1(2); 135-137.

6. Mayeux R, Ottman R, Maestre G, Ngai C, Tang CX, Ginsberg H, Chun M, TyckoB, Shelanski M. Synergistic effects of traumatic head injury and apolipoprotein-epsilon 4 in patients with Alzheimer's disease. *Neurology* 1995; 45(3 Pt 1): 555-557.

7. Holmes C, et al. Systematic inflammation and disease progression in Alzheimer's disease. *Neurology* 2009; 73(10): 768-774.

8. Perry VH, Newman TA, Cunningham C. The impact of systemic infection on the progression of neurodegenerative disease. *Nature Review of Neuroscience* 2003; 4(2): 103-112.

9. Hanning CD. Postoperative cognitive dysfunction. *British Journal of Anaesthesia* 2005; 95(1): 82-87.

10. Collins N, Blanchard M, Tookman A, Sampson E. Detection of delirium in the acute hospital. *Age & Ageing* 2010; 39(1): 131-135. DOI:10.1093/ageing/afp201

11. Majer M, et al. Association of childhood trauma with cognitive function in healthy adults: a pilot study. *Bio-Med Central Neurology* 2010; 10: 61.

12. Wang H-X, et al. Psychological stress at work is associated with increased dementia risk in late life. *Alzheimer's and Dementia* 2012; 8: 114-120.

13. Rissman RA, Staup MA, Roe A, Nicholas L, Kenner JJ, Rice C, Vale W, Sawchenk PE. Corticotropin-releasing factor receptor-dependent effects of repeated stress on tau phosphorylation, solubility, and aggregation. *PNAS* 2012; 109(16): 6277-6282. DOI: 10.1073/pnas.1203140109.

14. www.alzheimers.org.uk/site/scripts/news_article.php?newsID=1243

15. Yaffe K, et al. Post-traumatic stress disorder and risk of dementia among U.S. veterans. *Archives of General Psychiatry* 2010; 67(6): 608–613. DOI: 10.1001/archgenpsychiatry.2010.61.

16. Johansson L, et al. Midlife psychological stress and risk of dementia: a 35-year longitudinal population study. *Brain* 2010; 133: 2217–2224. DOI: 10.1093.

17. Whitehouse PJ, George D. *The Myth of Alzheimer's* USA: St Martin's Press; 2008.

Chapter 8

Physical and mental illness

It is sometimes difficult for people to understand that dementia is not a mental disease as such. This is particularly confusing because the diagnosis of dementia is most often (though not always) made by a psychiatrist. Research also shows that some forms of mental illness are risk factors for dementia.

Alzheimer's disease is a physical disease which affects the brain. Actual physical changes take place in the tissues of the brain which alter the way that the brain works. In the advanced stages of Alzheimer's disease, the atrophy of the brain can be measured. As far as is known, it is not the result of any other disease.

Vascular dementia is caused by changes in the circulatory and the vascular system which result in a lack of adequate blood supply to the brain. Some doctors think that a vascular 'event' such as a stroke may also trigger Alzheimer's disease (see chapter 1) and that the two forms of dementia are more closely connected than was previously thought to be the case.

These two diseases are the most common forms of dementia, although there are many other more rarely seen types which appear to develop as primary diseases.

At the same time, it is also known that there are many rare physical diseases that may lead to dementia, including progressive HIV/AIDS, Creutzfeldt–Jakob disease (CJD), supranuclear palsy, Korsakoff's syndrome, and Binswanger's disease. Some people with multiple sclerosis, motor neurone disease, Parkinson's disease or Huntington's disease may develop dementia as a result of the progression of one of these diseases.

Because we are used to modern medicine being able to treat many conditions, and even to cure some of them, and because in the developed world we no longer fear the scourges of the past such as contagious diseases and disease caused by poor sanitation, there is a tendency to see illness as something which has only a short-term effect and which, after a cure has been effected, will not leave any residual problem in the human body. People have tended to become quite blasé about even very serious illness, such as pneumonia. The need to convalesce is no longer considered necessary and even taking extra rest after an illness is slightly frowned upon as 'malingering' or making a fuss.

In fact all illness leaves its mark upon the body. People live longer now and medical practitioners are beginning to see the residual effects of illness manifesting itself in later life. For example, we now know that there is a connection between polio and symptoms of lassitude, weakness and muscle fatigue in later life, known as 'post polio syndrome'. The viral illness chickenpox, which many people contract as children, can resurface in later life as shingles, an extremely painful condition.

An analysis reported in the *Journal of Social Science and Medicine* examined whether childhood illness had a long-term effect on the appearance of chronic disease in later life. The authors reported that poor childhood health increases 'morbidity' (the likelihood of becoming ill) in later life. An association with poor health in childhood was found for cancer, lung disease, cardiovascular conditions, and arthritis/rheumatism. Non-infectious diseases were associated with higher rates of cancer and arthritis or rheumatism in later life, while infectious diseases were strongly associated with lung conditions, such as emphysema and bronchitis. The writers stated that: 'Our results point to the importance of an integrated health care policy based on the premise of maximizing health over the entire life cycle'.[1]

Such findings do not mean that we should be anxious about trivial illness or worry about past medical history. There is, however, ample evidence for making sure that we give our bodies time to recover after illness and that we make every effort not to allow neglect of our health to cause problems in later life.

We will see in the course of this chapter that some illnesses, both physical and mental, and some traumatic events predispose people towards dementia in later life. There are indeed chronic diseases and disorders which are known to have a 'connection' with dementia. The most well documented of these are cardiac and vascular disease (including stroke) and diabetes.

Stroke

Many people who suffer a stroke which causes temporary cognitive, as well as neurological, problems make a considerable, if not a full, recovery. They do not develop dementia and may go on to live comfortable and active lives. However, the fact is that suffering a stroke does increase your chances of developing dementia. **Atrial fibrillation** in someone who has suffered an **ischemic** stroke seems to be associated with an increased risk of developing dementia.[2] If you have a stroke and are discovered to suffer from atrial fibrillation, you will be offered medical treatment to reduce the chances of a further stroke.

Someone who has suffered a stroke will normally be subject to a number of tests and investigations to discover the ostensible cause. Health issues such as high blood pressure or cardiac disease will hopefully be addressed by the attending medical team. If you have had a stroke you can help yourself by making full use of all the physical therapy offered to you and by adopting a positive 'can do' attitude. Cognitive and physical recovery can happen over a number of months or years. The part of the brain which has effectively 'died' following the loss of blood supply will not recover (it is known as an **infarct**) but other parts of the brain may, and frequently do, take over the functions of the dead cells and remarkable recovery can be made.

There are two main types of vascular dementia known to be related to stroke: 'multi-infarct dementia' (MID) and 'single-infarct dementia'.

Multi-infarct dementia (MID) is the result of multiple, small strokes and is a common form of dementia. It develops when blockages in the blood supply to the brain occur frequently over a period of time in the smaller blood vessels, giving rise to many tiny and widespread areas of damage. These small strokes are commonly known as **transient ischaemic attacks** (TIAs). Often someone can suffer a TIA without any major symptoms and they may even be unaware that it has happened. Sometimes the only symptoms are fleeting, such as a few moments dizziness or a slurring of speech which rights itself in moments, or a weakness and numbness in a limb which passes off and may be put down to cramp or to sitting too long in one position. These continuing small strokes can go on for years, causing gradual loss of function and leading to confusion and intellectual deterioration. A feature of this type of vascular dementia is that some people experience periods of relative stability before another TIA causes further significant and abrupt worsening of the symptoms.

Single-infarct dementia results from a single stroke that is extremely severe or affects a particular area of the brain to which the damage is limited.

Sub-cortical vascular dementia (also known as 'small vessel disease related dementia') is a further form of vascular dementia. It is not caused by stroke but may be experienced by somebody who has also had a stroke. It is caused by injury to small blood vessels that are deep within the brain. The onset of this type of dementia is more gradual than stroke-related dementia, and so it appears more like the onset of Alzheimer's disease rather than the 'stepped' deterioration common to multi-infarct vascular dementia.

If you have suffered a stroke you can make every effort to recover your physical abilities, and making adjustments to your lifestyle and co-operating with medical teams will help to prevent further strokes. This will help to preserve your cognitive abilities.

If you have been diagnosed with vascular dementia (as a result of several minor strokes/TIAs, for example), you may be given medication aimed at preventing further strokes. Treatment of vascular dementia is aimed at preventing more damage and capitalising on the cognitive abilities which are retained. Therefore, the suggestions in the chapters on exercise, social and cognitive stimulation, and nutrition are all relevant.

You can reduce your risk of suffering a stroke by taking regular exercise, refraining from smoking and controlling your blood pressure. You cannot usually anticipate a stroke, although there is evidence that a transient ischaemic attack is a serious warning sign of stroke and should not be ignored.

Up to 40 per cent of all people who have experienced a TIA will go on to have an actual stroke. Most studies show that nearly half of all strokes occur within the first two days after a TIA. Within two days after a TIA, 5 per cent of people will have a stroke. Within three months after a TIA, 10 to 15 per cent of people will have a stroke. If you believe that you have suffered a TIA, you should see your doctor without delay.

Diabetes

Diabetes is an increasingly common health condition. There are 2.9 million people diagnosed with diabetes in the UK and an estimated 850,000 people who have the condition but do not know it.[3]

Diabetes is the term used for a condition where the amount of glucose in the blood is too high because the body cannot metabolise it properly. When the body is working as it should, the organ called the pancreas produces a hormone called 'insulin' that allows blood sugar (glucose) to enter the body's cells, where it is used as fuel. Problems arise when the pancreas either does not produce any insulin, or does not produce enough. It may also be that the body's response to insulin becomes gradually weaker so that the pancreas has to produce more and more insulin without it ever being enough; this is called 'insulin resistance'.

There are two main types of diabetes: type 1 (often called juvenile-onset diabetes because it usually develops in childhood) and type 2 (sometimes called maturity-onset diabetes). Type 1 diabetes develops when the insulin-producing cells in the body have been destroyed and the body is unable to produce any insulin. Type 2 develops when the body can still make some insulin, but not enough, or when the body is unable to use the insulin being produced.

Diabetes is a serious condition and should not be treated lightly. If uncontrolled, it can lead to problems with blood circulation which can affect the eyes, heart and peripheral parts of the body (hands and feet, especially fingers and toes).

A growing body of research links diabetes with both Alzheimer's disease and vascular dementia. There is even a school of thought which suggests that Alzheimer's disease is actually a third type of diabetes.[4]

Non-insulin dependent diabetes has specifically been identified as a significant risk factor for age-related cognitive impairment, cognitive decline and dementia.[5] It has been demonstrated that people with **mild cognitive impairment (MCI)** who also have diabetes are three times more likely to develop dementia than those who have MCI alone.[6] The term MCI is used to describe someone who has memory impairment but no impairment in other cognitive functions or problems with the activities of daily living. (For more information about mild cognitive impairment see chapter 2.) There is evidence that patients who have diabetes are more likely to suffer cognitive impairment following a stroke[7] than those patients who do not have diabetes.

If you refer to chapter 6, on nutritional factors and dementia, it becomes clear that the problem lies in the metabolism of glucose and the effect this has on the brain. The brain uses glucose as its sole food (although it cannot store glucose), making use of almost a quarter of the glucose and oxygen which the body takes in. Because the brain uses glucose as its main source of energy it might be thought that a high level of glucose in the blood would be good for the brain, making it work better. In actual fact, fluctuations in blood glucose level, such as are caused by a diet high in carbohydrate (which the body breaks down into glucose, its absorbable form) and sugar including the sugar found in fruit (fructose), are detrimental. The brain needs a sustained and balanced supply of glucose, and this is best obtained from eating foods which cause blood glucose levels to rise more slowly and to be sustained for longer. Uncontrolled diabetes can lead to excessive high and low levels of glucose.

What does this mean in terms of avoiding dementia? Firstly, the risk factors for maturity-onset diabetes are well known. Do not assume that because many people are developing the condition it is not serious. You should take strenuous steps to avoid becoming diabetic. Whilst some of the risk factors may not be under your control, others, like excessive weight gain, lack of exercise and high blood pressure are likely to be within your control. Further information about risk factors is readily available on the Diabetes UK website and in their literature.[3] Remember that, aside from the risk of dementia, diabetes increases the risk of experiencing many other health problems too.

If you have been diagnosed with type 2 diabetes, you may be able to reverse the process by losing weight and addressing other health issues. If this is not possible, take the condition seriously. Adjust your diet, attend for medical screening and take your doctor/diabetic nurse's advice.

Diabetics who have been diagnosed with early stage dementia need special attention from their carer to watch blood glucose levels and take medication in a timely manner.

Other physical conditions

A number of other physical conditions have been linked with dementia especially in people known to carry the ApoE4 gene (for further information about ApoE4 see chapter 2), but research into these is still ongoing. Information about some of these conditions and the current state of research is included here for those who are interested. It is important to remember that, because we do not know the actual cause(s) of dementia, some of these lines of research may later be proved not to be relevant.

Herpes simplex

Ruth F Itzhaki, from the University of Manchester, UK, has done a substantial amount of research which suggests that a common virus, the herpes simplex virus type 1 (HSV1), acting in combination with the APoE gene, may have a major causative role. This is the virus which causes the common cold sore. Ruth Itzhaki presents evidence that the virus is, indeed, a factor in Alzheimer's disease (AD). However, her research, published in the *Lancet*, cautions that: 'the combination of HSV1 in brain and carriage of an APOE-epsilon 4 allele [gene] is a strong risk factor for AD, whereas either of these features alone does not increase the risk of AD.'[8] In other words, you should not necessarily worry just because you are prone to develop 'cold sores'. Other factors may play a more important part in the possibility of developing dementia.

Age-related macular degeneration

Scientists have known for some time that there is a connection between Alzheimer's disease and age-related macular degeneration (AMD) – the deterioration of the part of the retina called the 'macular', which provides our central field of vision. This condition is a major cause of sight problems in older people.

One of the early signs of Alzheimer's disease is the presence of 'extracellular senile plaques' in the brain – deposits of a protein called **amyloid** that disrupt communication between brain cells. These plaques are akin to deposits of cellular debris that are responsible for age-related macular disease; they build up between the retina and choroid layers at the back of the eyeball and disrupt vision.

Because of these parallels, researchers were prompted to study the appearance of the two diseases together within a major population study, the 'Rotterdam study'. This study was set up in the Netherlands to investigate factors that determine the occurrence of cardiovascular, neurological, ophthalmological, endocrinological and psychiatric diseases in elderly people. In a paper published in the *American Journal of Epidemiology* the researchers reported that subjects who had advanced AMD when the study began showed an increased risk of developing Alzheimer's disease. Their conclusion was that the neural degeneration occurring in AMD and that in AD might have a common **pathogenesis**, or underlying disease process.[9] However, the association was only significant for the most severe stages of AMD and the authors pointed out that this depended also on smoking and atherosclerosis (hardening of the arteries). Smoking is an established risk factor for AMD. (For further information on research results connecting smoking with incidence of dementia, see chapter 3 on personality and lifestyle.)

Hearing impairment

Hearing impairment may seem a strange factor to associate with dementia. However, a piece of research published in 1989 found that *untreated* hearing impairment was more prevalent in those with dementia and that the risk of dementia increased with the degree of hearing loss. The researchers did point out that there was no suggestion that hearing loss was a cause of dementia; rather that hearing loss might reveal or exacerbate the symptoms. Hearing impairment can cause social isolation and can also contribute to a general loss of understanding of the environment as well as, perhaps, contributing to depression.[10]

People with dementia are often reluctant to wear hearing aids even when they have been prescribed and carers sometimes find it difficult to ensure that they are worn consistently. A person who has dementia who also has a severe hearing loss will be likely to be more confused if he/she cannot hear what is going on around him/her.

Infection

Along with the evidence around HSV1 (*Herpes simplex*), there is emerging discussion of the possibility of some forms of dementia (as well as other chronic conditions, such as heart disease) resulting from infection. *Chlamydophila pneumoniae* and several types of bacteria, collectively known as 'spirochetes', have been suggested as possible causes.[11] Evidence to date has been inconsistent, however.

Scientists at the University of Texas Medical School in Houston did some research which involved injecting brain tissue from a confirmed Alzheimer's patient into mice and compared the results with a control group. Those mice injected with the Alzheimer's brain extracts developed plaques and other alterations to the brain typical of Alzheimer's disease. This research raises the possibility that some cases of Alzheimer's disease may arise from an infectious process similar to diseases like Creutzfeldt-Jakob disease. [12]

What *is* known is that infections of any kind are likely to accelerate neurodegeneration in someone who has dementia or mild cognitive impairment. Urinary and chest infections, in particular, are known to exacerbate symptoms in people with dementia and there is a school of thought which believes that inflammation is the prime 'culprit' in the development of dementia, particularly inflammation caused by infections.

Systemic inflammation – inflammation of the whole body – is known to have direct effects on brain function. Recently a number of observational studies linked the intake of **non-steroidal anti-inflammatory drugs (NSAIDs)** with a lowered risk of developing Alzheimer's disease,[13] and for a while this looked like a very promising research route. Unfortunately, **randomised controlled trials** so far have not confirmed any beneficial effect from taking NSAIDs. However, scientists are still following up this line of research, and it is possible that a different dose than that used in the randomised controlled trials, or the use of NSAIDs at an earlier stage of disease or for a different length of time, might show benefit.

There are a number of (mostly rare) infectious and inflammatory conditions which can lead to dementia and that can be treated leading to the improvement or stability of any dementia symptoms. These diseases include Hashimoto's encephalitis, syphilis, Lyme disease (later stages) and HIV/AIDs. Usually other (non-dementia) symptoms will be evident and lead to a correct diagnosis and treatment.

Episodes of delirium, in which elderly and demented patients become extremely disoriented and confused, are frequently caused by infections, injury or surgery (see below). Urinary tract infections, which are usually caused by bacteria, appear to be particularly common inducers of psychiatric symptoms which can sometimes mimic dementia.

Post-operative cognitive impairment

Following an operation under general anaesthetic some people develop a severe (and temporary) form of confusion often termed post-operative delirium. It is known that people who suffer post-operative delirium are more likely to suffer from dementia at a later date.[14] This has been noticed more particularly in patients undergoing coronary bypass grafting. For more detail on post-operative cognitive impairment see chapter 7 on trauma.

Physical disease as a trigger

Clearly physical disease and the risk of dementia are not unconnected. Whilst not suggesting that you should become over-concerned about minor illness, the evidence implies that as we grow older we should take care of our physical health, be sensible about minor infections or injuries, and not allow minor health problems to become major ones through self-neglect. If you have a long-standing health problem you should not become blasé about the way you manage it. Whilst the human body has huge recuperative powers, you should respect the potential for future damage and protect against this as far as possible.

The family and carers of people who have been diagnosed with dementia often state that they date the appearance of symptoms from a severe illness, the beginning of a physical health problem or a stay in hospital for a surgical operation. Some doctors tend to dismiss this anecdotal evidence, suggesting that there is no robust research which proves such incidents precipitate early symptoms of dementia. Others, including consultant psychiatrists who specialise in elderly care, are more cautious. If you notice symptoms of cognitive loss following a major physical illness or surgical intervention, do not allow yourself to be dismissed as neurotic.

Other causes of memory loss and confusion

It is important to remember that there are some physical problems – one example is a vitamin B12 deficiency – which may cause memory problems and mild confusion. When people present to their doctor with suspected dementia, the doctor will normally conduct tests to screen out the possibility of such a cause. If you are worried about the possibility of a vitamin deficiency you can check this with your doctor.

There are also some drugs, or combinations of drugs, which may cause these symptoms. Sometimes the symptoms may arise even after you have been taking the drug for some time without problems.

Memory loss and confusion do not always mean dementia. If you suspect a deficiency or a drug interaction you should mention this to your doctor or pharmacist. Pharmacists are often more knowledgeable about drug interactions than GPs.

Depression

Depression is linked to dementia and often accompanies the diagnosis, although it is not clear whether the depression is part of the illness or is caused by the diagnosis. Many of us might consider that such a diagnosis might make us depressed. It is also not clearly understood whether depression precedes the development of dementia or is a causal effect. Depression is particularly common in people diagnosed with vascular dementia or with dementia due to Parkinson's disease.

Most of the symptoms of depression are generally well known. They include feelings of hopelessness and sadness, loss of interest in daily activities, feelings of worthlessness and possibly guilt, feelings of isolation, loss of appetite and difficulty with sleeping, problems with concentration and decision making, and tiredness and loss of energy.

You may recognise from chapter 2 that many of these symptoms are similar to those experienced by someone with dementia. Indeed, it is not uncommon for someone who has dementia and retains insight to believe that they are suffering from a form of depression and to visit the doctor believing this to be their problem. It is unfortunately quite common for people actually to be treated for depression for some time before the possibility of a diagnosis of dementia is considered, especially in people under the age of 65.

****

I believed that my difficulties in concentrating and my confusion were because I was depressed. I put this down to the fact that I had recently retired and that two close friends had died in the past six months. Initially I felt a little better when I was given an anti-depressant medicine but the confusion and memory problems did not get better. It was almost a relief to have a proper diagnosis and at this point my GP explained that I was probably suffering from depression alongside the dementia.

****

Josh Woolley and colleagues studied the likelihood of those with emerging dementia being diagnosed initially with depression or other psychiatric problems. Their investigation involved 252 patients with a neurodegenerative disease diagnosis seen between 1999 and 2008. Of these, 28.2 per cent (nearly a third) had received a prior psychiatric diagnosis. Depression was the most common in all groups, but those with **fronto-temporal dementia** received a psychiatric diagnosis more often than those with Alzheimer's disease. The researchers concluded that dementia is often misclassified as psychiatric disease, with patients that had behavioural-variant fronto-temporal dementia at highest risk of misdiagnosis. The authors of this paper pointed out that the study could not rule out the possibility that psychiatric disease is an independent risk factor for dementia (see more research below). However, if misdiagnosed, then patients may receive 'delayed, inappropriate treatment and be subject to increased distress'.[16]

Depression can make the behavioural symptoms of someone suffering from dementia worse, and treating the depression will mean that both the person with dementia and his/her carers will be better able to cope, although some medical opinion suggests that conventional anti-depressant treatment does not work to lift depression in those with dementia.

There are a number of links between clinical depression during adulthood and dementia in later life but it is difficult to draw definite conclusions. Robert S Wilson, PhD, of Rush University Medical Center, Chicago, and colleagues, studied 917 older Catholic nuns, priests and monks who did not have dementia, beginning in 1994. Those with more symptoms of depression at the beginning of the study were more likely to develop Alzheimer's disease. For each depressive symptom registered at the beginning of the study, the risk of developing Alzheimer's disease increased by an average of 19 per cent, and the annual rate of cognitive decline increased by an average of 24 per cent. In this study, those who developed Alzheimer's disease did not show any increase in depressive symptoms in the period just before the diagnosis was made. These researchers therefore concluded that symptoms of depression might be associated with changes in the brain that reduce its resistance to dementia.[17]

Looking at the connection another way, research reported in the *European Journal of Epidemiology* suggests that there may be a genetic link between a susceptibility to depression and a higher than normal risk of dementia.[18] In this study of 6596 subjects, researchers looked at the association of self-reported depression which required treatment by a psychiatrist, to family history of psychiatric disease, dementia and Parkinson's disease. Not surprisingly perhaps, a family history of psychiatric disease was significantly associated with overall depression. In addition, people who had two or more first-degree relatives, such as parents, siblings or children, with dementia had a higher risk of depression. Those with only one relative with dementia had no increased risk. The researchers suggested that this study indicates that there might be 'shared susceptibility gene(s) underlying these diseases'. Of course it might be concluded that the stress of caring for two or more relatives with dementia could be a cause of depression.

Depression, and additionally bipolar disorder, are also associated with a higher than average risk of dementia in another piece of research which looked at all hospital admissions for primary affective disorder (low mood and depression) in Denmark during 1970–1999. A total of 18,726 patients with depressive disorder and 4248 patients with bipolar disorder were included in the study. Risk of a later diagnosis of dementia was significantly increased according to the number of times patients had been admitted to hospital previously. It was calculated that every admission for depression increased the possibility of later dementia by 13 per cent and every admission for bipolar disorder increased the possibility of dementia by 6 per cent. The researchers concluded that the risk of later dementia increased with the number of episodes of hospitalisation with depression.[19]

This is not an easy conclusion to interpret, however. Is one to conclude that hospital admission makes dementia more likely or that a more severe experience of bipolar disorder (therefore involving hospital admission) is the risk factor?

Mood disorders in general may be risk factors for the development of dementia. A study involving 455 people with mood disorders, including major depression and bipolar disorder, compared with 1003 'normal' controls, showed that cognitive decline developed faster in people with mood disorders after the age of 65 than in the control group. The authors concluded that not only might depression in later life be an early manifestation of dementia but that those who develop depression or fail to recover from an earlier depression may have a higher risk of developing dementia. The researchers did, however, point out that the results could equally show that changes resulting from past disease or injury might cause both mood disorders and dementia.[20]

This sample of the research into a possible causal link between dementia and depression indicates both the difficulties which researchers encounter and the lack of robust conclusions from research to date. The only clear conclusion appears to be that there is some connection between clinical depression and a later diagnosis of dementia. Clinicians also know that people diagnosed with dementia are often also depressed.

Schizophrenia

Schizophrenia is a mental illness characterised by a breakdown in thought processes and by poor emotional responsiveness. It commonly manifests itself as 'hearing voices' (auditory hallucinations), paranoia, strange delusions, and disorganised patterns of speech and thought, and it is accompanied by significant social and/or occupational dysfunction. It is a completely different disorder from dementia and the onset of symptoms generally occurs in young adulthood.

Some research has been done on the connection of an extracellular matrix protein which may be involved in the pathologic changes in both schizophrenia and Alzheimer's disease.[21] The cells which secrete this protein are reduced in the brain of someone with schizophrenia and they are also reduced in the brain of someone with Alzheimer's disease. As with Alzheimer's disease though, the causes of schizophrenia are unclear. Where dementia develops in people with schizophrenia it seems to be similar to fronto-temporal dementia[22] (see chapter 2).

Recently a particular study has been made of the association of the drug benzodiazepine with the development of dementia. Benzodiazepine is primarily used for treating the symptoms of anxiety and sleep disorders over short periods. It is widely prescribed in developed countries. It is known that the drug impairs free recall and the recognition of information. Studies focusing on the association between benzodiazepine use and dementia or cognitive decline in elderly people have previously shown conflicting results. Some found an increased risk of dementia or cognitive impairment in benzodiazepine users,[23, 24] whereas others reported a potential protective effect.[25]

In 2012 a large, prospective, population-based study of elderly people who were free of dementia and did not use benzodiazepines until at least the third year of follow-up was reported in the *British Medical Journal*. This research concluded that new use of benzodiazepines 'was associated with a significant, approximately 50% increase in the risk of dementia'. The researchers reported that this result remained stable after adjustment for potential confounding factors, including any cognitive decline before starting benzodiazepine and clinically significant symptoms of depression.[26]

Precautions

If you have been diagnosed with any form of dementia, or if you are caring for someone with dementia, you should remember that it is a serious disease. In the early days, especially, there are often no obvious physical signs and people are apt to forget how serious the condition is. If you have dementia you should consider that your immunity is compromised. Every effort should be made to protect someone with dementia from catching infections, even such minor things as the common cold, and especially such illnesses as chest and urinary infections. If any elective surgery is required it should be carefully planned and efforts should be made to ensure that the person with dementia reaches the hospital in the best possible state of physical health. Sometimes doctors themselves do not appear to take these precautions seriously so it is up to carers to do their best. Keep people with colds away from a person with dementia, take colds seriously and do your best to make sure that no complications develop. Any infection may result in a (sometimes temporary) worsening of dementia so be aware of this.

If the person you care for suffers from diabetes you should make absolutely certain that his/her blood sugar is kept regulated. People with dementia (even if previously self-medicating) may forget to check their blood sugar levels and to take their medication or may become confused about time and dosages. Unregulated blood sugar levels will cause a person with dementia to become more confused and disorientated.

If the person you are caring for has vascular dementia you should familiarise yourself with the symptoms of small stroke (TIA) and be alert for any signs of this; a deterioration in cognitive ability may result.

If the person you are caring for has been prescribed medication such as anti-depressants or mood-controlling drugs, and once they have been stabilised on these drugs, you should not discontinue or reduce (or increase) the dose without checking with the doctor first, even if you think the medication is causing other symptoms. The doctor can help to find the dose which will give most benefit with the least side effects. Discontinuing or giving medication erratically can make someone's symptoms worse.

Key points

- Illnesses and traumatic events may pre-dispose people to dementia

- Some rare diseases may lead to dementia in their later stages

- Diabetes is a major risk factor for cognitive dysfunction and dementia

- Cardiac and vascular disease are a fundamental factor in vascular dementia

- Some other diseases increase the chances of a later diagnosis of dementia

- Some research has shown a possible infectious cause of Alzheimer's disease

- Depression frequently accompanies dementia

- People with dementia should be protected as far as possible from infections

References

1. Blackwell DL, Hayward MD, Crimmins EM. Does childhood health affect chronic morbidity in later life? *Social Science & Medicine* 2001; 52(8): 1269–1284.

2. Mizrahi EH, Waitzman A, Arad M, Adunsky A. Atrial fibrillation predicts cognitive impairment in patients with ischemic stroke. *American Journal of Alzheimer's Disease and Other Dementias* 2011; 26(8): 623-626. DOI: 10.1177/1533317511432733.

3. Information from Diabetes UK http://www.diabetes.org.uk

4. Zhao WQ, De Felice FG, Fernandez S, et al. Amyloid beta oligomers induce impairment of neuronal insulin receptors. *FASEB Journal* 2008; 22: 246-260.

5. Logroscino G, Kang JH, Grodstein P. Prospective study of type 2

diabetes and cognitive decline in women aged 70-81 years. *British Medical Journal* 2004; 328(7439): 548-503.

6. Velayudhan L, Poppe M, Archer N et al. Risk of developing dementia in people with diabetes and mild cognitive impairment. *British Journal of Psychiatry* 2010; 196(1): 36-40.

7. Mizrahi EH, Waitzman A, Blumstein T, Arad M, Adunsky A. Diabetes mellitus predicts cognitive impairment in patients with ischemic stroke. *American Journal of Alzheimer's Disease and Other Dementias* 2010; 25(4): 362-366. DOI: 10.1177/1533317510365343.

8. Itzhaki RF, et al. Herpes simplex virus type 1 in brain and risk of Alzheimer's disease. *Lancet* 1997; 349(9047): 241-244.

9. Klaver CCW, et al. Is age related maculopathy associated with Alzheimer's disease? *American Journal of Epidemiology* 1999; 150(9): 963-968.

10. Uhlmann RF, et al. Relationship of hearing impairment to dementia and cognitive dysfunction in older adults. *Journal of the American Medical Association* 1989; 261(13): 1916-1919.

11. Ewald PW. *Plague Time: The new germ theory of disease*. Anchor Books; 2002.

12. Morales R, et al. De novo induction of amyloid-B deposition in vivo. *Molecular Psychiatry* 2012; 17: 1347–1353. DOI: 10.1038/mp.2011.120.

13. In 't Veld BA, Ruitenberg A, Hofman A, et al. Nonsteroidal anti-inflammatory drugs and the risk of Alzheimer's disease. *New England Journal Medicine* 2001; 345: 1515-1521. DOI: 10.1056/NEJMoa010178.

14. Hanning CD. Postoperative cognitive dysfunction. *British Journal of Anaesthesia* 2005; 95(1): 82-87.

15. Holmes C, et al. Systemic inflammation and disease progression in Alzheimer disease. *Neurology* 2009; 73(10): 768-774.

16. Woolley JD, Khan BK, Murthy NK, Miller BL, Rankin KP. The diagnostic challenge of psychiatric symptoms in neurodegenerative disease: rates of and risk factors for prior psychiatric diagnosis in patients with early neurodegenerative disease. *Journal of Clinical Psychiatry* 2011; 72(2); 126-133.

17. Wilson et al. Depressive symptoms, cognitive decline, and risk of AD in older persons. *Neurology* 2002; 59(3): 364-370. DOI: 10.1212/WNL.59.3.364

18. Fahim S, et al. A study of familial aggregation of depression, dementia and Parkinson's disease. *European Journal of Epidemiology* 1998; 14(3) 233-238. DOI: 10.1023/A:1007488902983

19. Kessing LV, Andersen PK. Does the risk of developing dementia increase with the number of episodes in patients with depressive disorder and in patients with bipolar disorder? *Journal of Neurology Neurosurgery and Psychiatry* 2004; 75: 1662–1666. DOI: 10.1136/jnnp.2003.031773

20. Gualtieri CT, Johnson LG. Age related cognitive decline in patients with mood disorders. *Progress in Neuro-Psychopharmacology & Biological Psychiatry* 2008; 32(4): 962-967; 0278-5846.

21. Aoki T, Mizuki Y, Terashima T. Relation between schizophrenia and Alzheimer's disease: the reelin signalling pathway. *Psychogeriatrics* 2005; 5: 42-47.

22. de Vries PJ, Honer W, Kemp P,McKenn P. Dementia as a complication of schizophrenia. *Journal of Neurology Neurosurgery and Psychiatry* 2001; 70: 588-596.

23. Gallacher J, Elwood P, Pickering J, Bayer A, Fish M, Ben-Shlomo Y. Benzodiazepine use and risk of dementia: evidence from the Caerphilly Prospective Study (CaPS). *Journal of Epidemiology and Community Health* 2012; 66: 869-873.

24. Wu CS, Wang SC, Chang IS, Lin KM. The association between dementia and long-term use of benzodiazepine in the elderly: nested case-control study using claims data. *American Journal of Geriatric Psychiatry* 2009; 17: 614-620.

25. Fastbom J, Forsell Y, Winblad B. Benzodiazepines may have protective effects against Alzheimer disease. *Alzheimer's Disease and Associated Disorders* 1998; 12: 14-17.

26. Billioti de Gage S, Bégaud B, Bazin F, Verdoux H, Dartigues J-F, Pérès K, Kurth T, Pariente A. Benzodiazepine use and risk of dementia: prospective population based study. *British Medical Journal* 2012; 345: e6231.

Chapter 9

If you are worried that you are developing dementia

What should you do if you think you are developing dementia?

Many, if not most, of us have worried at some time that we are developing cognitive problems. Perhaps it is an increase in those 'senior moments'. Maybe we find that we just cannot grasp how to work a new piece of household equipment. Possibly our family and friends are suggesting that we may have a problem and ought to see a doctor.

The popular press is not helpful in the way it describes the first symptoms of dementia. It is common to see statements such as 'dementia begins by forgetting small things such as where we have put our keys'. But forgetting where we have put our keys is not in itself an indication of early dementia. If you are a carer and have read chapter 2 in this book, you should have a clearer idea of what dementia is and what it is not and be able to decide whether your worries warrant further investigation.

Look again at these symptoms:
- Short-term memory loss
- Impaired judgement
- Difficulties with abstract thinking
- Faulty reasoning
- Inappropriate behaviour
- Loss of communication skills
- Disorientation as to time and place

- Gait, motor and balance problems
- Neglect of personal care and safety
- Hallucinations, abnormal beliefs, anxiety, agitation.

Unfortunately, not everyone in the early stages of dementia is able to understand or realise that they have a problem with **cognition**. Dementia by its very nature can prevent the clear thinking and analysis of symptoms which might help this realisation. You may think that your memory is fine. Everyone forgets the odd appointment, don't they? It is part of getting old. You have not forgotten where you put your wallet. Obviously someone must have moved / stolen it.

If you are not sure whether you have a problem, or if someone close to you is suggesting that you do, you might first like to look at these questions and answer them honestly:

- Does it seem that the person closest to you (wife/ husband / child) is less patient than they used to be?
- Do people accuse you of forgetting appointments? (even if you are sure you did not make the appointment)
- Do you sometimes find that things you use have disappeared from their usual place?
- Do you ever find yourself somewhere without remembering how you got there?
- Do complete strangers say hello and suggest you were ignoring them?
- Do you feel that you cannot be bothered to do anything?
- Do you lose track of the time quite often?

No one wants to think that they are suffering from a serious disease. Doctors' surgeries are full of patients who did not attend early in their illness because they hoped that by ignoring the symptoms they would go away. For this reason, if your family or friends are saying they are worried about your memory, you should take their concerns seriously. It might help to remember that other conditions can cause memory loss and confusion. You may not have dementia. However, if you do have the early stages of dementia it is better to have the diagnosis as soon as possible so that you can get all the support available.

Your first step should be to make an appointment to see your GP. If a family member has said that he/she is worried about you, it is a good idea to take him/her along with you when you go to the GP. Your relative will be able to explain to the doctor why he/she is worried about you.

Your doctor is likely to do some physical tests, such as blood tests. This is because there are some illnesses not connected with dementia which can affect your cognition and your memory. Most of these illnesses are treatable so you should welcome the chance to see if a specific illness is the cause of your cognitive problems.

It is quite likely that the doctor will administer a short 'mental test'. This is simply to check whether the problems you and/or your relative are referring to are 'normal' for your age and state of health. You should not be worried about the test and you should not think of it in terms of passing or failing.

After these tests, if the doctor thinks that you have a cognitive problem which needs further investigation, he/she is likely to refer you to a psychiatrist who specialises in mental health in older people. Occasionally he/she may refer you to a geriatric consultant instead. If you have private medical insurance and wish to use that you will probably be referred to a consultant neurologist. The consultant (neurologist, psychiatrist or geriatrician) is likely to give you a longer mental health test and will spend some time talking to you and discussing any problems which you are having with memory. He or she is also likely to want to have a private discussion with your relative, be it wife/husband, or son or daughter – whoever has most to say about your present problems. This can be quite difficult as it may seem as though people are 'talking behind your back', but you should bear in mind that no one wishes to hurt you. It is easier for relatives to speak about things which they have noticed when you are not present to be hurt or upset or even surprised by what may be said.

After the first appointment, the consultant may refer you for yet further tests, perhaps with a psychologist, or he/she may order a brain scan. Finally, you will meet the consultant again and hopefully receive a diagnosis. If the diagnosis is not clear to you, then you should ask any questions you need to at this stage.

Some doctors are reluctant to give a clear diagnosis. A diagnosis of dementia depends upon signs of a progressive cognitive decline. Sometimes it may be necessary for the consultant to see you again after a few months to assess if this is happening in your case. It can be difficult to 'wait and see', but the consultant will be trying to do his/her best to give you an accurate diagnosis. In the meantime, there is nothing to prevent you doing things to help yourself and if you read further in this chapter you can find out what those things are.

If you are diagnosed with early stage dementia or **mild cognitive impairment**, or if you are caring for someone in this situation, is there anything you can do which can help? Throughout this book I have referred to research which indicates a causal effect for dementia and which has highlighted actions which can help to slow down the effects. In each chapter you will find short sections on how you can help yourself or someone close to you if there is a diagnosis of dementia. The following information is given here so that either you, if you have dementia (or mild cognitive impairment), or your main helper (generally referred to as 'the carer') can work out what is best for you.

1. Give medication a try

After a diagnosis you should consider accepting any medication you are offered, at least for a trial period. Many people are put off by the mention of side effects. Modern-day protocols mean that doctors have to point out the possible side-effects of any drug they prescribe. This does not necessarily mean that you will suffer these side effects. Medication comes with an explanatory leaflet which details side effects and also the likelihood of these occurring. If 10 per cent of people are likely to have side effects, this means that 10 out of every 100 people who take the drug will suffer them. It also means (perhaps more importantly) that 90 out of every 100 people who take the drug will *not* suffer side effects. Most of the dementia drugs are given at a lower dose first, partly to allow for monitoring of side effects. Your doctor should explain this to you.

The reason for at least trialling medication is that, limited in effect as these drugs are, they are the best solution that medicine can offer at the present time. Remember that dementia is progressive; it does not go away or get better on its own. If you refuse dementia drugs, you are refusing the only specific medical treatment that is available. If you do suffer from side effects, they may only last for a short time, or the doctor may be able to adjust your dose to minimise them. If the worst comes to the worst, you can stop taking the medication, but it is worth giving it a try.

Not everyone can be offered the medication that is available as there are some contra-indications (health reasons why someone should not take the medicine). Your doctor will explain these to you if they apply. If he/she does not explain, you should ask why you are not being prescribed medication. Since most of the dementia drugs are now 'off licence', they are comparatively cheap and should be freely available where there is no medical reason to indicate otherwise.

2. Accept support

Accept any support that is offered to you. In many areas, consultant psychiatrists and geriatricians work closely with support workers from the Alzheimer's Society, or with dementia advisers, and they will offer you a referral to one of these for support. There will, in any case, be a Community Mental Health team of psychologists, nurses, occupational therapists, speech and language therapists and, sometimes, social care workers, who can give ongoing support where this is required. Sometimes people who are referred privately to a consultant neurologist may miss out on this support because they are not referred, so you should be aware that it is available and make enquiries about how you obtain this.

Often in the first stages after diagnosis people are reluctant to accept 'outsiders' and have a strong belief that they can manage the illness alone. This is very understandable. Be aware though that the support is on offer and make a note of contact details in case you want to reconsider later. Even if you have refused support in the past, workers from the Alzheimer's Society will happily help you when you do approach them. It is also your right to have ongoing support from NHS professionals and social care even if you have refused this support previously. Support workers from the Alzheimer's Society can help you to get access to social care support.

If you get the chance to talk to other people who have dementia or are looking after someone who has dementia they will probably recommend that you accept any support you can get.

3. Increase (or keep up) exercise

Help yourself – or help the person you care for. Exercise is known to help maintain cognitive levels. In the chapter on exercise we saw that one theory is that exercise has an effect on brain plasticity. In an animal study using rats and mice given the opportunity (but not forced) to use an exercise wheel, researchers focused on a chemical called 'brain-derived neurotrophic factor' (BDNF) because this makes possible neuronal connectivity. In simple words, this factor allows neurons to connect to one another and change their connections when new skills are being learned. The researchers expected that the response to exercise would be restricted to motor sensory systems of the brain, such as the cerebellum, primary cortical areas or basal ganglia. Amazingly, after several days of voluntary wheel running, increased levels of BDNF were found in the rats and mice's hippocampus, a part of the brain normally associated with higher cognitive function. The hippocampus plays important roles in the consolidation of information from short-term memory to long-term memory, and in spatial navigation. In Alzheimer's disease, the hippocampus is one of the first regions of the brain to suffer damage; memory problems and disorientation appear among the first symptoms of the disease. This research indicated that exercise actually strengthens the neural structure helping the neurons to make connections with each other.[1]

One large-scale US study, in which levels of exercise and cognitive impairment status were measured over a 10-year period, showed not only that exercise had a beneficial effect on cognition but that the number and different types of exercise performed were inversely associated with the onset of cognitive improvement. The interesting point is that whilst exercise of any kind was found to be beneficial, the number of different types of exercise made a difference. Those engaging in four different types of exercise over a two-week period decreased their risk (of cognitive impairment) when compared with those who engaged in one type of exercise.[2]

This information, described at greater length in chapter 5 on physical exercise, is repeated here as an example of research which has shown that exercise is beneficial if you have been diagnosed with MCI or dementia. Physical exercise is thought to be more beneficial even than so-called 'brain exercise'. In some cases, it may seem that the body subconsciously knows that exercise is beneficial. Some people with dementia become very restless and start to take long walks or to pace up and down indoors. Sometimes it seems that they cannot settle down to rest. There may seem to be an inexplicable urge to keep on the move. Others find that they lose the urge for physical activity. It may seem too much effort to even get up from the chair.

There are many ways to increase the amount of exercise you undertake. You can increase the amount you walk – for example, walking to the shops or round the local park. You can work in the garden. Digging, mowing the grass and weeding are all good examples of bodily exercise. You could re-start a hobby such as swimming or golf which you have allowed to lapse. If your mobility is restricted you can take exercise classes aimed at those with mobility problems.

If you are caring for someone with dementia it may be that you have to provide encouragement and opportunity for exercise. Do not be put off by the notion that you are 'nagging'. Remember that in encouraging more exercise you are acting in the best interests of the person you care for. Exercise is always more enjoyable if it is done along with someone else. Many forms of exercise are also an opportunity to improve your social contacts.

4. Keep up social activities

Exercise your brain and keep up a varied social life. It is easy to believe that by completing our favourite crossword each day we are 'exercising the brain', and indeed this is a useful as well as enjoyable thing to do. However, to really keep the brain active, we need to keep it on edge by trying new experiences, visiting a variety of places and making the effort to enjoy the company of others. Retirement is a wonderful opportunity to try new experiences. People with dementia may find it quite stressful to plan new things and to visit new places so it may be up to relatives and friends to take over the planning and organising of outings, trips and holidays. Be assured that it is good for someone in the early stages of dementia to keep up their social life and to have new experiences, but be aware also that they will need extra reassurance in strange situations and that they may need someone with them to help them easily to find their way around.

Encourage friends to continue to visit by being open about the diagnosis and giving them information about dementia if they need it. Keep up attendance at any regular outings, such as church services or social clubs, sports occasions and hobby groups, visiting your adult children and attending local events. By all means do crosswords, quizzes and word searches, and if you are already a competent computer user, try playing computer games. There is some evidence that playing electronic games helps the brain. It is probably better not to put yourself under stress by trying to learn something completely new, so if you are not used to the computer do not attempt to learn now. However, you could certainly revisit old hobbies and pastimes to see if they reinvigorate you. Above all keep doing the things that you enjoy as long as you are able to do so.

If you are the carer, then be aware that you may have to take quite an active part in encouraging a continued social life. You may have to initiate activities and visits, and sometimes this can be quite tiring, especially if the person you are helping seems less than enthusiastic. It helps to enlist the assistance of friends here. Explain to them the effect that dementia has on the 'executive' part of the brain and ask them to give invitations or to suggest outings and to persist in the face of perceived inertia.

5. Look after your physical health

Guard yourself against infection and accidents. This does not mean that you should become fearful and over cautious, but you should, if you have a diagnosis of dementia or are caring for someone who has a diagnosis, take sensible precautions against catching cold. You should nurse a cold so that it does not develop into a secondary infection, practise good hygiene and eat a sensible diet to give your body the best chance to fight an infection. If you think that you have any infection, then visit your doctor promptly for the proper treatment. If you are caring for someone with dementia, remember that any infection can make cognitive problems worse, and be alert if the person you care for seems suddenly to go 'downhill'. It may be the first signs of an infection or illness. Urinary tract infections, for example, can take you by surprise in this way. If your GP is not sympathetic or seems not to understand the problems of having or caring for someone with dementia, then remember that it is your right to change your GP at any time.

Check your home environment and make sure that simple things like poor lighting, trailing wires and loose rugs are attended to in order to minimise the chance of falls. Don't take unnecessary risks when doing odd jobs around your property. Use the proper safety equipment and tools for the job, and don't climb up ladders or on to furniture to reach things without someone else being at hand. You want to avoid any chance of a stay in hospital because an accident which results in a hospital stay may make dementia worse.

An admission to hospital (perhaps due to an accident) is very likely to result in a deterioration in dementia symptoms. Records show that 30 per cent of elderly people admitted to hospital end up being discharged into a residential care home.

6. Eat a good diet

Eat a good nourishing diet. Remember that the diet that was recommended in mid-life may not suit an older person with dementia. It is more important to increase your intake of fat and oily fish than to struggle to eat 'five a day'. You should reduce your intake of processed carbohydrates and try to eat as much unprocessed food as possible. You should cut sugar intake and be careful about the amount of alcohol you drink.

If you are caring for someone with dementia, remember that they may forget how many drinks they have had and you may need to help them to keep account of their alcohol intake.

There is some research which indicates benefit from various food supplements and taking these is unlikely to do any harm and may be beneficial. It is important to ensure a proper intake of vitamin D and vitamin E and you might like to try adding coconut oil to your diet. If someone with dementia starts to lose weight, then it is most important to ensure that everything eaten is rich in nutrients. In this case you should switch to using full cream milk, increase your intake of cheese and eggs, and cut down on cakes, biscuits and sweet things so that you are hungry for nutrient-rich food. Food can also be fortified to help increase the nutritive value, and your speech-and-language therapist or dietician (if you have one) can advise you about this.

7. Attend to practical matters without delay

Attend to practical matters about the future. Presently we do not have a cure for dementia, and we know that it is a progressive disease. If you have just been diagnosed with dementia, then take the opportunity to deal with practical matters whilst you are able. It is worth sitting down with your family and discussing your own needs and wishes for the future. If you become unable to manage your financial affairs, you would wish them to be managed by someone you can trust. Set up a Lasting Power of Attorney now if you haven't already done so and then this can be arranged easily should it become necessary. Do not leave this until you 'need it'. The time when you need to arrange this is now whilst you can still think clearly.

If someone with a diagnosis of dementia is living alone then it is important to think carefully about future arrangements. As the disease progresses, people who have dementia find it more difficult to deal with the activities of daily living, such as washing or bathing, dressing, preparing meals and keeping the house clean. Although someone who lives alone can be helped initially by arranging for visiting carers, and for friends or neighbours to be on hand to help, this kind of arrangement is limited. As the disease progresses, it will be difficult for someone with dementia to continue to live alone and independently. The early days after a diagnosis are an opportunity for family and friends to help them to plan arrangements for the future.

8. Do not hide your condition

Do not feel that you have to 'cover up' or, as someone once put it to me, 'avoid going public' about the diagnosis of dementia. If people know that you have a problem, they can help out. They are also more likely to keep offering invitations and to continue social contact if they understand what is wrong. It can be very frustrating for friends to have their invitations turned down or their visits curtailed without understanding why. In these circumstances it is understandable that acquaintances fall away and friends become more distant. If you are caring for someone with dementia, the time will come when you will be glad of any help and be grateful for friends who continue to keep up a relationship, even when their overtures are rejected by the person with dementia.

It is a good idea to make sure that friends and neighbours understand about the diagnosis and also what they can do to help. Most people are pleased to help, but many do not understand how they could adapt their behaviour or how dementia can affect a person's cognitive abilities. The Alzheimer's Society offers some very clear explanatory factsheets which you can download from their website and pass around if you feel unable to explain clearly yourself.

9. Avoid family conflict

Relatives should be aware of the difficulties that can arise within families when one of their members is diagnosed with dementia. Differences of opinion in how to manage certain behaviours, practical decisions that have to be made, and a basic misunderstanding of what dementia means, can cause huge and surely unnecessary rifts in families, which may persist for years. Where there is a second or subsequent marriage and step-children are involved, life can become even more complicated. It is a very good thing if, early in the days after the diagnosis, the family can get together and agree to act only in the best interests of the person with dementia. This can mean setting aside old resentments about favouritism during childhood, feelings of betrayal after a divorce and subsequent re-marriage, and feelings of guilt or anger at the amount of extra care being given, or in some cases not given, by others. None of this is easy to do but it can help to think about whether you actually want to make the life for the person diagnosed as happy and stress-free as possible. Sons or daughters who are not regular visitors to the home should beware of suggesting that:

'Dad seems fine to me.'

Or

'You're making too much of it, Dad. Mum seems to be managing most things.'

The truth is that unless you are on the spot every day you cannot understand the level of stress which a carer may be going through as the disease progresses. What children *can* do is to provide relief and respite. Parents are often reluctant to ask children to help under the mistaken surmise that they are too busy or should not be asked to interrupt their routine. Dementia is generally a disease of older people and their children may be at a very busy time of their lives, occupied with their careers or with a growing family. It is worth remembering that as the disease progresses, carers need literally 'time off'. People with dementia often do not like being left alone – they seem to need the security of having someone around them. Later in the progression of the disease, it may be unsafe to leave someone who has dementia alone as they may no longer recognise common dangers; they may forget ordinary safety routines, or to eat and drink, and they may wander off looking for their carer. Adult children can give real respite by giving their time to allow Mum to visit the hairdresser, Dad to tackle his garden in peace, either parent to go for a quiet game of golf or visit the cinema or simply have a couple of hours out with friends. Even a few hours 'off' each week can make the difference between a carer managing to cope and collapsing from over-stress.

Children should also be understanding about the possible future need for residential respite care. Unless they are prepared to 'take over' the caring role for 24 hours a day, for at least a week, they can have no concept of the need the main carer may have for a 'holiday' from 24-hour care.

10. Don't make major life changes

Try to avoid making major life changes – for example, moving house. It is important that the person with dementia feels secure and one of the things that enhances this sense of security is familiarity with one's surroundings and avoiding major changes. Often, when confronted with the diagnosis, families think this is the right moment to make changes which they have been meaning to make 'sometime in the future'. This may be, for example, downsizing to a smaller home or even considering moving to a 'retirement complex.' On the surface this may seem a good idea since it is wise to plan for a future when extra help and support may be needed. A garden or a house which is becoming too large to manage, for example, can seem like an extra unnecessary burden. It is also true that some retirement complexes offer assisted living as part of their package and this may seem attractive when considering the future. However, house moves, even sensible ones, are stressful and disruptive to routine and generally after the move the person with dementia becomes worse, seeming to be more insecure and to lose more abilities more quickly than expected. The family home, especially, can be a source of many memories, and old memories play a big part in giving a person with dementia a feeling of security and continuing identity. If you can arrange help in the house and garden for the things you can no longer manage, and (if necessary) organise transport if you can no longer use the car, then it may be better to continue living in familiar surroundings as long as possible.

11. Make the most of 'now'

It may seem that a diagnosis of dementia is a devastating blow and perhaps the advice above has given you a great deal to think about. But this time can also be an opportunity to take stock and remember the important things in life. If you have been diagnosed with dementia, or if you are caring for someone with dementia, then by all means prepare for the future – but above all, *now* is the time to enjoy the present. Get the most out of life every day.

Key points
- Onset of dementia is not simply 'memory problems'
- Someone with dementia is unlikely to recognise that they have a problem
- People who are worried should first see their GP
- If you have a confirmed diagnosis you can help yourself by following advice in this chapter
- Family, neighbours and friends can help, especially if they understand the problems

References

1. Cotman CW, Berchtold NC. Exercise: a behavioural intervention to enhance brain health and plasticity. *Trends in Neoroscience* 2002; 25: 295-301.
2. Jedrziewski MK, et al. Exercise and cognition: Results from the National Long Term Care Survey. *Alzheimer's and Dementia* 2010; 6(6): 448-455. DOI: 10.1016/j.jalz.2010.02.004.

Appendix I

The brain – a simple description with reference to dementia

The following description of the brain – its structure and function – has been included here to aid understanding of the physical changes that take place in the various conditions that underlie dementia. It is not intended by any means to be comprehensive, even at a simple level.

The first thing to note is that the brain consists of a number of interrelated structures and of different types of cells, and that these different parts are responsible for different aspects of activity and behaviour. For this reason, the symptoms of disease will depend upon which parts of the brain are affected.

The brain consists of three main sections: the hindbrain, the midbrain and the forebrain. The hindbrain and midbrain are mainly concerned with basic life support functions, such as blood pressure and respiration. The forebrain is responsible for the majority of higher brain functions, such as memory and language.

The human brain is larger than that of any other mammal in relation to body size. As already stated, it is made up of many specialised areas that work together. These include:

- **The cerebral cortex** – this is the outermost layer of brain cells. Thinking and voluntary movements begin in the cortex.
- **The brain stem** – this lies between the spinal cord and

the rest of the brain and controls basic functions like breathing and sleep.

- **The basal ganglia** – these are a cluster of structures in the centre of the brain. They coordinate messages between many other brain areas.
- **The cerebellum** – this is at the base and the back of the brain. It is responsible for coordination and balance.

The cerebral cortex

The part of the brain we are most concerned with in this book is the cerebral cortex. In humans this is a thick layer of neural tissue that covers most of the brain. This layer is folded in a way that increases the amount of surface that can fit into the volume available. Interestingly, in humans the portion of the cerebral cortex devoted to vision is greater than in any other mammal.

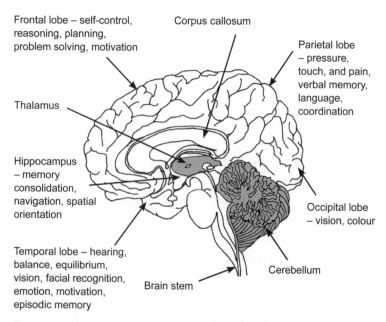

Frontal lobe – self-control, reasoning, planning, problem solving, motivation

Corpus callosum

Parietal lobe – pressure, touch, and pain, verbal memory, language, coordination

Thalamus

Hippocampus – memory consolidation, navigation, spatial orientation

Occipital lobe – vision, colour

Temporal lobe – hearing, balance, equilibrium, vision, facial recognition, emotion, motivation, episodic memory

Brain stem

Cerebellum

Figure 1: Vertical cross-section through the brain

The cortex is divided into two 'hemispheres' (right and left) and each hemisphere is then further divided into four 'lobes': the occipital lobe, parietal lobe, temporal lobe, and frontal lobe. (However, be aware that some classification systems are slightly different and may include more 'lobes'.) Within each lobe are numerous cortical areas, each associated with a particular function. The left and right sides of the cortex are broadly similar in shape, and most cortical areas are replicated on both sides. Some areas, though, show strong 'lateralisation' (that is, the specialist centre is only, or mostly, on the left or the right side of the brain). This is particularly true of the areas that are involved in language. In most people, the left hemisphere is 'dominant' for language, with the right hemisphere playing only a minor role. There are other functions, such as spatio-temporal reasoning, for which the right hemisphere is usually dominant.

Each hemisphere of the brain interacts primarily with one half of the body, but for reasons that are unclear, the connections are crossed: the left side of the brain interacts with the right side of the body, and vice versa. Motor connections from the brain to the spinal cord, and sensory connections from the spinal cord to the brain, both cross the midline at the level of the brainstem. The two cerebral hemispheres are connected by a very large nerve bundle called the 'corpus callosum', which crosses the midline above the level of the structure known as the thalamus (see Figure 1), which is responsible for relaying sensory and motor signals to the cerebral cortex. There are also two much smaller connections, known as the 'anterior commissure' and the 'hippocampal commissure', as well as many subcortical connections that cross the midline. The corpus callosum is, however, the main avenue for communication between the two hemispheres. It connects each point on the cortex to the mirror-image point in the opposite hemisphere, and also connects to functionally related points in different cortical areas.

The occipital lobes receive input from the visual pathways and damage in this area will result in loss of vision or loss of part of the visual field. It may also result in an inability to identify colours or to recognise words. It is believed that this lobe has other functions also. This means that where the occipital lobes are damaged in someone with dementia, he/she could have difficulty seeing what an object is, despite both eyes being in perfect condition.

The parietal lobes are located in the middle section of the brain and are associated with processing tactile sensory information, such as pressure touch, and pain. A portion of the brain known as the 'somatosensory cortex' is located in these lobes and is essential to the processing of the body's senses. Damage to the parietal lobes can result in problems with verbal memory, an impaired ability to control eye gaze and problems with language. Following damage to the parietal lobes, people may suffer an impairment of their ability to identify objects by touch, clumsiness on the side of the body opposite to the damage, neglect of one side of the body, distortion of body image and an inability to draw or follow maps or to describe how to get somewhere. Tasks such as reading and writing, which require putting letters and words together, and calculation, which involves ordering and combining numbers, are critically dependent on the dominant (left or right) parietal lobe. This dominant side has also been heavily implicated in a condition known as 'apraxia' (an impairment of learned purposive movements). People with dementia often have problems with simple sequential actions like getting dressed. This is caused both by losing the memory of the movements required for dressing (such as fastening a button or pulling up a zip) and by a lack of coordination; the underlying problem is in the parietal lobes.

The temporal lobes are located near the temple on each side and are concerned with hearing, balance and equilibrium. They also contribute to some of the more complex aspects of vision, such as the ability to recognise faces. The temporal lobes also play a part in emotional and motivational behaviours and are involved in memory. In people with Alzheimer's disease, it is the episodic memory (the collection of past personal experiences that occurred at a particular time and place) that is most commonly damaged. It is not yet clear exactly how or where long-term memories are stored, or if they are 'stored' at all,[1] but it is thought that memories are made by strengthening the connections between relevant nerve cells. Some remote or distant memories, perhaps of childhood experiences, are apparently stored more deeply or are more available to recall than less familiar or recent memories, such as what one did yesterday. It is possible that they are more deeply entrenched in the mind because important events have been re-remembered many times over the years, and so are more rehearsed than recent memories. This is why some people with dementia may find it easier to discuss certain often-recalled aspects of their childhood than what has happened that day or even a few minutes before.

The frontal lobes are associated with executive functions, such as self-control, planning, reasoning and abstract thought. They are also responsible for problem solving, judgement and motor function. Damage to these lobes causes people to lose their initiative and results in a failure to inhibit socially unacceptable impulses. The middle portion of the frontal lobes generates our motivation and general impetus. If this part of the brain is affected, people can lose their 'get up and go', or executive function, becoming lethargic and reluctant to get out of bed or perform particular activities. They may become unable to begin an action, even a familiar one. Sometimes, if the action is started for them (for example, if someone else guides their hand holding a tooth brush) they may carry on the action. Carers often regard this type of loss of initiative as laziness, but it is a direct consequence of the loss of cells in this area of the brain.

Damage to these areas may also result in impairment to some aspects of memory. For the sufferer, it can be like being a learner all over again. Many multi-stage tasks, such as cooking and shopping, become very difficult because the pattern, or plan of action, gets lost during the processing. Damage to the frontal lobes can also cause people to get 'stuck' on what they are doing. (This is known as 'perseveration'.) As the frontal lobe interacts with many other brain areas, this perseveration may take the form of using the same word over and over again, or taking one piece of clothing out of a wardrobe and then removing all the other clothes without a specific reason. Sometimes people with damage in this area may continually move things from place to place without any obvious purpose.

The cells that make up the brain

The brain is composed of many different types of cell, but the primary functional unit is a cell called a **neuron** (see Figure 2). All sensations, movements, thoughts, memories, and feelings are the result of signals that pass through neurons. Neurons have a cell body which contains the nucleus, **dendrites** which extend out from the cell body like the branches of a tree and receive messages from other nerve cells, and **axons** from which signals travel away from the cell body, either down to another neuron, a muscle cell, or cells in some other organ. Some cells are wrapped around the axon to form an insulating sheath. This sheath can include a fatty molecule called myelin, which provides insulation for the axon and helps nerve signals travel faster and farther.

The place where a signal passes from one neuron to another is called the **synapse**. When the signal reaches the end of the axon of one neuron, it stimulates tiny sacs to release chemicals known as **neurotransmitters** into the synapse. The neurotransmitters cross the synapse and attach to receptors on a nearby cell. If the receiving cell is also a neuron, the signal can continue the transmission to the next cell.

An individual neuron may change in several ways during

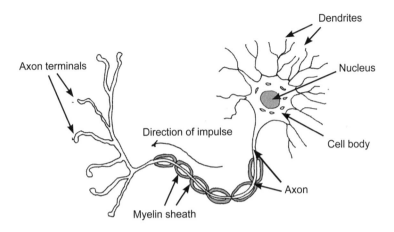

Figure 2: A nerve cell, or 'neuron'

learning. For example, a neuron may increase its release of its transmitter, or it may have increased responsiveness to stimulation.

One neurotransmitter, acetylcholine, is called an 'excitatory neurotransmitter' because it generally makes cells more able to work. It governs muscle contractions and causes glands to secrete hormones. Alzheimer's disease is associated with a shortage of acetylcholine. This shortage means that signals are transmitted less easily between neurons.

The hippocampus

The hippocampus is the part of the brain that is involved in memory formation, organisation and storage. It is a structure that is particularly important in forming new memories and connecting emotions and senses, such as smell and sound, to memories. The hippocampus is a horseshoe-shaped, paired structure, with one half located in the left brain hemisphere and the other in the right hemisphere. The hippocampus acts as a memory indexer by sending memories out to the appropriate part of the cerebral hemisphere for long-term storage and re-trieving them when necessary.

The hippocampus is involved in several functions of the body, including consolidation of new memories, emotional responses, navigation and spatial orientation.

Atrophy of the hippocampus is common in Alzheimer's disease. The hippocampus may also be affected in small vessel disease (vascular dementia). These are the two most common types of dementia.

It is impossible to say for certain which areas of the brain will be affected most in which order for each individual with dementia. Everyone's brain is unique and the way in which each person develops and uses his/her brain is unique to them. This also explains why each individual may show different symptoms at any one point in the manifestation of the disease. Each person will have a complex set of difficulties and experi-ence. Some people lose the ability to speak coherently early on, whilst others can continue to be able to hold a good conversation even though they may need help with dressing, bathing or other activities of everyday living. Some people become disorientated, losing a sense of direction, early on but retain the ability to carry out familiar tasks. Most people do show signs of short-term memory loss, but some people can carry on living independently for a while using memory 'aids' to help with this. Many people with dementia have problems with their vision which are not apparent during normal eye examinations. This is because the part of the brain which interprets what the eye 'sees' is damaged.

In a few forms of dementia there are specific indications of the brain area affected. For example, in frontotemporal dementia, damage is usually focused in the front part of the brain. At first, personality and behaviour changes are the most obvious signs, and memory problems may not be so obvious.

Diagnostic tests

The tests which doctors use for diagnosis, and later to assess the value of any drug treatment, are meant to look at the different brain areas and the way in which these may be damaged. However, doctors themselves agree that these tests are not necessarily entirely accurate. They are indicative, and a drop in the test 'score' is useful to indicate a possible disease progression.

Reference

1. Fernyhough C. *Pieces of Light: the New Science of Memory.* Profile Books, 2012.

Appendix II

Useful sources of further information

Alzheimer societies in the English-speaking world

Alzheimer's Society
Tel: +44 (0)20 7423 3500
Website: www.alzheimers.org.uk

Alzheimer's Research UK
Tel: +44 (0)1223 843899
Website: www.alzheimersresearchuk.org/

Alzheimer Society of Ireland
Tel: +353 (01) 207 3800
Website:www.alzheimer.ie

Alzheimer's Scotland
Tel: +44 (0)808 808 3000
Website: www.alzscot.org

Alzheimer's Australia
Telephone: +61 1800 100 500 (helpline)
Website: www.fightdementia.org.au

Alzheimer Society Canada
Tel: +1 416-488-8772
Website: www.alzheimer.ca

Alzheimer's Association (USA)
Tel: +1 800-272-3900
Website: www.alz.org

Alzheimer's Disease Education and Referral (ADEAR) Center
Tel: +1-800-438-4380 (toll-free)
Website: www.nia.nih.gov/alzheimers

Dementia societies

Dementia Research Centre
Tel: +44 (0)20 3448 4773
Website: www.ucl.ac.uk/drc

Dementia UK
Tel: +44 (0)20 7874 7200
Website: www.dementiauk.org/

Sources of support

Age UK
Tel: +44 (0)800 169 6565 (advice line)
Website: www.ageuk.org.uk

Carers Trust
Tel: +44 (0)844 800 4361
Website: www.carers.org

Carers UK
Tel: +44 (0)808 808 7777
Website: www.carersuk.org

Diabetes societies

Diabetes UK
Tel: +44 (0)20 7424 1000
Website: www.diabetes.org.uk

Diabetes Australia
Tel: + 61 (02) 6232 3800
Website: www.diabetesaustralia.com.au

Canadian Diabetes Association
Tel: +1 416-363-3373
Website: www.diabetes.ca

American Diabetes Association
Tel: +1-800-342-2383 (helpline)
Website: www.diabetes.org

Down's syndrome societies

Down's Syndrome Association
Tel: +44 (0)845 230 0372
Website: www.downs-syndrome.org.uk

Down Syndrome Australia
Tel: +61 (02) 9841 4444
Website: www.downsyndromensw.org.au

Canadian Down Syndrome Society
Tel: +1-800-883-5608
Website: www.cdss.ca

National Down Syndrome Society (USA)
Tel: +1-800-221-4602 (helpline)
Website: www.ndss.org

Glossary

ADAS-Cog – The most commonly used test for the symptoms of dementia and their relative progression. It consists of 11 tasks measuring problems with memory, language, learning, attention and other cognitive abilities.

Alzheimer's disease – The most common cause of dementia, characterised by *gradual* decline in mental processes, generally starting with disorientation, short-term memory loss and loss of motivation. The brain characteristically shows plaques of the protein **amyloid beta** and **neurofibrillary tangles**.

Amyloid beta – A protein (peptide) that is essential to normal brain functioning but which is thought to cause Alzheimer's disease by building up into insoluble 'plaques' in the brain.

Amyloidosis – A condition where amyloid proteins are abnormally deposited in organs or tissues and cause harm.

Amino acids – Organic chemicals which mix in various combinations to make protein.

ApoE genes – ApoE is the abbreviation for 'apolipoprotein E', an essential body protein that is managed by the ApoE gene, found on human chromosome 19. The gene comes in three forms: 2, 3 and 4. ApoE4 is associated with a higher than average risk of developing dementia. As our chromosomes come in pairs, we all have two chromosome 19s and therefore, two ApoE genes. Those of us with two ApoE4s have the highest risk. Those with one ApoE4 and one ApoE2 or ApoE3 come next.

Astrocytes – Characteristic star-shaped cells found in the brain and spinal cord.

Atrial fibrillation – An erratic (fast and irregular) heartbeat.

Axon – A long slender projection from a nerve cell which carries electrical impulses away from the nerve body.

Beta amyloid plaques – see **Amyloid beta**.

Borderline histrionic – Excessively emotional with attention-seeking behaviour, including an excessive need for approval and inappropriately seductive behaviour.

Case-control study – Research where each participant receiving the active intervention (or attribute) being studied is matched by a 'control' participant who is similar in all respects other than the intervention or attribute being studied.

Cholesterol – A fatty substance known as a 'lipid' that is vital for the normal functioning of the body. It is mainly made by the liver, but can also be found in many foods that we eat. Cholesterol is needed everywhere in the brain as an antioxidant and to manufacture the neurotransmitters, such as acetylcholine, by which nerve cells communicate.

Chromosome – An organised structure of DNA and protein found in the nucleus of each living cell. Humans have 23 pairs of chromosomes, each of which consists of genetic coding and other regulatory material that together encodes the development of the individual.

Chromosome 21 – The chromosome that is associated with Down's syndrome. As a result of faulty cell division, the single cell from which a new individual will grow starts out with three copies of the

21st chromosome rather than the usual pair. All cells in the body are derived from this first cell and will all consequently have an extra chromosome 21.

Cognition – The mental processes, including attention, memory, language production and understanding, problem solving, planning and decision making.

Cognitive reserve – The resistance of the mental processes to damage from trauma and/or disease.

Dementia – An umbrella term for the group of symptoms that characterise more than 60 different conditions, of which Alzheimer's disease is the most common.

Dementia with Lewy bodies – Dementia where the brain shows tiny spherical deposits (Lewy bodies) that develop in nerve cells, interrupting the action of chemical messengers.

Dementia pugilistica – Dementia that results from a blow, or many blows, to the head and is particularly associated with boxing.

Dendrites – Thread-like extensions of brain cells (neurons) that connect to other neurons and develop with learning.

Dissocial – Unfriendly to society; selfish; overlooking the rights of others.

Double-blind trial – see **Randomised controlled trial**.

Essential fatty acids – These are fats that the body needs to manufacture healthy cells and **prostaglandins** and which the human body cannot make for itself but must acquire from its food. These fats are omega-6 (linoleic acid) and omega-3 (alpha linolenic).

Fronto–temporal dementia – An umbrella term for dementias arising from damage to the frontal lobes of the brain, including Pick's disease, frontal or temporal lobe degeneration, and dementia associated with motor neurone disease.

Gene – A single element in the coding found in each cell in the body that dictates how that cell, and hence the whole person, should develop.

Hippocampus – A part of the cortex of the human brain that is responsible for consolidating short-term memory as long-term memory, and for spatial organisation. It is one of the first parts of the brain to be affected in Alzheimer's disease. Its name relates to its shape; 'hippos' is the Ancient Greek for 'horse', and 'campus' for 'sea monster' – in other words, 'sea horse'.

Hydrogenated fats – These are fats, such as vegetable oil, that would naturally be liquid at room temperature but by a process called 'hydrogenation' have been rendered solid. They are sold as 'spreads' and also used by food manufacturers in biscuits and other confectionary. There is increasing concern about their potential impact on health.

Infarct – Death of body tissue due to shutting off the blood supply, as for example in a stroke.

Intervention trial – Any research where a study is made of the effect of an 'intervention' (it could be a drug or some other sort of treatment, such as an exercise programme) on a group of individuals.

Ischaemia – A decrease in the blood supply to a bodily organ, tissue, or part caused by constriction or obstruction of the blood vessels by a blood clot.

Ketones – One of a group of organic compounds produced during the metabolism of fats.

Lewy body dementia – see **Dementia with Lewy bodies**.

Mild cognitive impairment (MCI) – Cognitive impairment, especially short-term memory loss, beyond what would be expected given age and education, but which is not significant enough to interfere with the activities of everyday living.

Mini-Mental State Examination (MMSE) – A 30-item questionnaire that is used to screen for impairment to mental processes and to assess decline in mental processes over time. It also called the 'Folstein test'.

Myelin – The fatty substance that forms a covering 'sheath' around the **axons** of nerve cells and facilitates the passage of electrical impulses through those cells.

Narcissistic – Excessive love or admiration for oneself.

Neural reserve – Spare capacity in the brain, in the shape of nerve cells, multiple linkages between nerve cells, and networks, that allows the brain to compensate for the effects of disease, trauma and aging.

Neurofibrillary tangles – Aggregations of a protein called 'tau' that are the primary markers, along with **amyloidosis**, in the brain of Alzheimer's disease.

Neuron – Nerve cells that make up the brain, spinal cord and peripheral nervous system. They consist of a cell body, containing the cell nucleus, a long tail (the **axon**) and many branching connections (**dendrites**) to other neurons.

Neuroplasticity – The brain's ability to reorganise itself by forming new neural connections throughout life.

Neurotransmitters – Chemical substances released from nerve endings to transmit impulses to other nerve cells (**neurons**). They include adrenaline (now generally called 'epinephrine'), dopamine and serotonin.

Non-steroidal anti-inflammatory drugs (NSAIDs) – A class of drugs, such as aspirin and ibuprofen, that provide pain relief, reduce fever and, at high doses, reduce inflammation, but are not steroids.

Paranoid – Exhibiting or characterised by extreme and irrational fear or distrust of others; unduly suspicious.

Pathogenesis – The process that leads to the development of a disease.

Placebo-controlled – see **Randomised controlled trial**.

Plaques – See **Amyloid-beta**.

Prostaglandins – Hormone-like substances present in tissues and body fluids that act as important chemical messengers or mediators. Unlike hormones, which are produced by specialised organs in the body, prostaglandins are produced, and act, locally.

Randomised controlled trial – This describes research that is carried out in a way that is regarded as the gold standard in clinical science, especially for assessing the efficacy of new treatments. 'Randomised' refers to the fact that participants in the trial ('subjects') are randomly allocated to either the treatment group or the 'control' group; they are not deliberately chosen for one or the other. 'Controlled' refers to there being equal numbers of active subjects (who receive the new drug, for example) and 'controls' who receive an imitation of the drug (a 'placebo'). If a trial is also described as 'blinded', or 'double-blinded', this means that neither the participants nor the researchers know who has been allocated to receive the active intervention or the placebo.

Schizoid – Extremely shy or reclusive with a lack of interest in personal relationships.

Spirochetes – Spiral shaped bacteria that lack a rigid cell wall and move by means of muscular flexion.

Synapse – The minute gap between the nerve endings of one **neuron** and those of another, across which neurons communicate by passing **neurotransmitters** from one to another.

Transient ischaemic attacks (TIAs) – Sometimes called 'mini strokes', these are episodes when insufficient blood reaches the brain for such a short time it is barely noticeable, though the effects may be similar to those of a full scale stroke.

Vascular dementia – Dementia that arises from problems with the supply of blood to the brain, typically from a series of **infarcts**. It is characterised by a stepped decline in mental processes, and is the second most common form of dementia.

Index

acetylcholine, 25, 88, 90, 163
    alcohol and, 43
ADAS-Cog, 79, 97, **169**
aerobic exercise, 75–76, 80–81, 84
affective (mood) disorders, 134–135
Age UK, 167
age-related macular degeneration,
    127
aging
    cognition and, 63
    normal vs abnormal signs and
symptoms, 14–17
agreeableness, 35
alcohol, 7, 41–45, 101–102
alpha-linolenic acid, 90, 94
aluminium, 100–101
Alzheimer's disease (AD), 119
    acetylcholine shortage, 88, 163
    age-related macular degenera-
tion and, 127
    aluminium and, 100–101
    definition, **169**
    depression and, 60, 132, 133
    diet and, 92
        exercise and, 80
    distinction from other dementias,
2–3, 13
    Down's syndrome and, 50, 51
    early-onset, 4, 18–19, 112
        education in, 56
    genetics *see* genetic factors
    medical treatment, 27–28

    physical development, 24–25
    schizophrenia and, 135
    smoking and, 40, 41
    vascular dementia mixed with,
25
    vascular 'events' and, 6, 65, 75,
108, 119
Alzheimer's Disease Assessment
    Scale-cognitive subscale
    (ADAS-Cog), 79, 97, **169**
Alzheimer's Research UK, 166
Alzheimer's societies outside
    England, 166–168
Alzheimer's Society (UK), 152, 166
    help and support from, 28–29
American Diabetes Association, 168
amino acids, 89, 97, **169**
amyloid beta (beta-amyloid), 50–51,
    169
    diets lowering levels of, 96
    Down's syndrome and, 50–51
    plaques *see* plaques
amyloid precursor protein (APP), 4,
    18, 19
amyloidosis, 92, **169**
anaesthesia, cognitive impairment or
    delirium following,
    108–109, 130
antioxidants, 90, 92, 99
apolipoprotein E/ApoE (and the
    gene), 4, 20, 40, **169–170**
    ApoE2, 20, **169–170**

Note: bold indicates references in the glossary section. Abbreviations: AD, Alzheimer's disease.

Note: bold indicates references in the glossary section. Abbreviations: AD, Alzheimer's disease.

Index

Note: bold indicates references in the glossary section. Abbreviations: AD, Alzheimer's disease.

Note: bold indicates references in the glossary section. Abbreviations: AD, Alzheimer's disease.

Index

Note: bold indicates references in the glossary section. Abbreviations: AD, Alzheimer's disease.

Note: bold indicates references in the glossary section. Abbreviations: AD, Alzheimer's disease.

Index

Note: bold indicates references in the glossary section. Abbreviations: AD, Alzheimer's disease.

Note: bold indicates references in the glossary section. Abbreviations: AD, Alzheimer's disease.

182